UW-W LIBRARY

MANUAL FOR THE APHASIA PATIENT

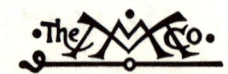

THE MACMILLAN COMPANY
NEW YORK · CHICAGO
DALLAS · ATLANTA · SAN FRANCISCO
LONDON · MANILA

BRETT-MACMILLAN LTD.
TORONTO

Manual for the Aphasia Patient

Mary Coates Longerich, Ph.D.

Speech Pathologist

College of Medical Evangelists, School of Medicine, Los Angeles, California

Foreword by J. M. Nielsen, M.D.

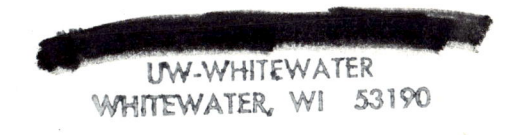

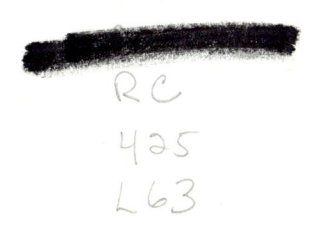

THE MACMILLAN COMPANY, NEW YORK, 1958

© *Mary Coates Longerich 1955, 1958*

All rights reserved—no part of this book may be reproduced in any form without permission in writing from the publisher, except by a reviewer who wishes to quote brief passages in connection with a review written for inclusion in magazine or newspaper.

First printing, March, 1958

Printed in the United States of America

ACKNOWLEDGMENTS

The author is grateful to J. M. Nielsen, M.D., and to Robert C. Robb, M.D., for the reading of the manuscript and for the helpful suggestions they have made; to Eugene G. Lindsay, D.D.S., for the drawings in Part Three; to her secretary, Marianne B. Lindsay, for her assistance in preparing and typing the manuscript; to Joyce B. Baisden, M.A., Charles H. Cramer, M.A., and her mother, Mayme Surber Coates, for editing the proofs.

M.C.L.

FOREWORD

Doctor Longerich has thoroughly shown her understanding not only of aphasia but of the aphasia patient. She has now met a need, long felt, of a guide for the aphasic and for members of the aphasic's family.

The member of the family who assists the patient with his aphasia therapy should be a person in whom the individual has confidence. Because the aphasic is often unable to assimilate a large amount of material during a therapy session, it is advisable that the relative work with the patient for short sessions (five or ten minutes) several times a day.

Some patients following their cerebral accident experience considerable spontaneous recovery, providing Nature gives them enough time and their health is otherwise adequate; whereas other patients, because of their severe brain damage, may not even be amenable to therapy. Naturally this book applies only to those patients who can benefit from aphasia therapy.

Since a large percentage of families may not be accessible to an aphasia therapist and since many may be unable to afford such services, this book should answer a real need.

J. M. Nielsen, M.D.

CONTENTS

Acknowledgments   v
Foreword, by J. M. Nielsen, M.D.   vii
Introduction   x
Part One: THE FAMILY HELPS THE APHASIC   1
Part Two: THE THERAPIST HELPS THE APHASIC   7
   A. Planning Aphasia Therapy   7
   B. Preparing the Muscles for Speech   17
   C. Imitating Lip and Tongue Movements   20
   D. Writing   22
   E. Help with Individual Sounds   26
   F. Suggested Readings   27
Part Three: DRILLS FOR THE PATIENT   29
   A. Drills for Receptive Aphasia   31
   B. Drills for Expressive Aphasia   169

INTRODUCTION

Manual for the Aphasia Patient is written primarily for the patient, his therapist, and his family. Part One deals with what the family can do to help the aphasic; Part Two pertains to specific techniques which the aphasia therapist can use; Part Three consists of actual drills for the patient.

Although Part One is directed particularly to the family, it contains important suggestions for all persons dealing with the aphasic. Hence it is advisable that the therapist read Part One in its entirety before embarking upon the therapeutic procedures of Parts Two and Three.

The entire manual is based upon the principles as outlined in the aphasia text, Longerich and Bordeaux, *Aphasia Therapeutics* (The Macmillan Co., New York, 1954). It is therefore important that the therapist study the text carefully before attempting to use this manual with the patient.

part one
THE FAMILY HELPS THE APHASIC

"My husband had a stroke almost six months ago, and he still isn't doing much talking. About all he can say is *yes* or *no*. Most of the time he gets mixed up on those words too. He may say *yes* when he actually means *no,* or *no* when he means *yes*. We're continually trying to find out what he wants. And he's so irritable. He cries a lot and seems to get upset at the least little thing. He's grouchy and doesn't seem to have any consideration for the children and me anymore. In fact, he just seems to have lost interest in everything—himself and us too! What can we do?"

Perhaps you have already asked this question about a member of your own family. You say he seems to be able to hear even the slightest sounds but he doesn't seem to understand what you say to him. This is often the case. In fact, most aphasics have some problem in understanding what they hear. However, in many cases the loss in this realm is only slight.

You ask what you can do to help this person. Fortunately, there is much you can do. Naturally this will depend on just how severely and in which areas the brain has been damaged.

If it has been at least six months since the time of his attack, it is probable that he has made the maximum amount of *spontaneous* recovery that could be expected. His further progress will depend largely upon just how much specific help he can be given. It is vitally important for the patient to have aphasia therapy just as soon as possible after the accident, injury, or stroke; for, during these early months, he will benefit more than at any other time.

How can you aid in his speech rehabilitation? First, you and other members of the family can do everything possible to make the patient feel accepted and wanted. Strive to make him aware that you approve of him *as he is*. This is important because he may feel so frustrated and helpless that he may hate himself and want to give up. When you talk with him, try to make him feel you enjoy being with him. Show this by your action and tone of voice. Never take the attitude that you're doing him a favor by showing him attention.

It is important also that you visit with the patient and help him to be relaxed in his surroundings. Husband, wife, sister, brother, son, or daughter—everyone in the family circle must strive to make him feel contented. Help him become aware that all of you are working as a team to assist him in his recovery. Such cooperation will aid him to develop a desire to help himself. This is important because the patient must *want* speech if he is going to make much headway in learning to talk.

In addition to helping the patient to be relaxed in his surroundings, there are numerous other things that will help him:

1. When talking with the patient, pronounce your words clearly and understandably. Every time you speak to him, you are setting for him a speech example—either good or bad.
2. If the patient's language immediately prior to the onset of the aphasia is different from the language he spoke as a child, he may revert to the language he used in early childhood. This frequently happens and should be no cause for concern. For example, if he

spoke German as a boy, he may after the attack say *nein* for *no, ja* for *yes, Tisch* for table, etc. Be pleased if he can get his idea across to you. Later on, when he shows an inclination to use the English words, help him with them.

3. Maintain a calm attitude whenever you are with the patient. If he frets or fumes, say something like, "It is understandable that you feel this way. We all get upset at times. Perhaps we can do_____to help work this out." At this point try to suggest some solution to the frustrating problem, in order to make him feel more relaxed. The patient will usually begin to calm down as soon as you start agreeing with him and showing him you understand why he should feel upset. Usually he will be more agreeable to a reasonable suggestion after you show him you're on his side, and that you're pulling *for* him—not against him.

4. Avoid frustrating the patient by such remarks as: "Now you can say *hello.* You said it yesterday, so you can say it now!" Frequently a patient may be unable to utter a word which he may have said just a few minutes previously. Few adults like to be treated like a child. If he feels like saying *hello,* he'll try.

5. Encourage the patient to take part in family activities. The goal is to help him to want to participate in life so that he will not tend to sit back and watch the world go by.

6. If you have any feelings of resentment toward the patient, he will quickly sense your attitude. First, therefore, go somewhere else and "blow off steam"; then try to be understanding of his mistakes, his errors, and his inability to say what he wants.

7. Endeavor to interest him in some hobby. Usually it is more helpful if it is an activity in which you can participate with him. You will find many helpful suggestions for hobbies in M. Ickis' *Pastimes for the Patient* (A. S. Barnes & Co., New York, 1945).

8. Frequently, the aphasia patient doesn't seem to be interested in anyone but himself. This display of self-centeredness is not to be looked upon as selfishness. He is now having a real problem in thinking abstractly; hence it is necessary and desirable for him to focus all his energies on solving his own problems first.

9. If it seems difficult for him to meet new or strange situations, avoid forcing them upon him. Similarly, if he appears shy and does not want to see or visit with certain relatives, show no concern. He is reacting in this way because he probably feels inadequate to meet the social situation. Try to follow his wishes and strive to make him feel happy in his surroundings.

10. Should the patient become angry or depressed because of his inability to say what he wants to say or do what he wants to do, avoid criticizing or scolding him. Instead, try to help him make his wants known. Ask simple, direct questions which he can answer with *yes* or *no.* As mentioned earlier, the patient frequently gets confused in indicating what he means. That is why you must be alert to discover just what he is trying to tell you.

11. Frequently, a patient may repeat a certain word, phrase, or activity over and over. Avoid making an issue over this intense desire to repeat, but strive to get him interested in something else.

12. If he shows lack of good judgment in making decisions, avoid getting impatient. Try to suggest various alternative decisions from which he can choose.

13. When with people, the aphasia patient sometimes is unable to control his laughter. Avoid scolding him but suggest some other activity which permits him to get away from the group until he calms down. Similarly, a patient may cry easily. Avoid being oversolicitous.

© *Mary Coates Longerich 1955, 1958*

Say something like, "We understand. All of us have our difficult times." Then try to lead him into another interest or activity.

14. If he tends to forget where he put things or how to perform certain activities, help him to realize you understand this problem and that you want to help him solve it.

15. If he is an adult—treat him as an *adult*. Causing him to feel he is acting like a child is most annoying to him. He will either rebel or withdraw into his shell. Remember, the aphasic has not lost his speech because he consciously wanted to lose it. He is in a frustrating situation, and he is probably trying his best to cope with it.

16. The patient may be unable to manage his bladder and bowel functions or may forget about telling you when he needs to go to the bathroom. Never scold him for such slips. It only upsets the patient and may cause him to withdraw into himself, even to the point of losing all desire to help himself.

17. In case he has an accident and spills something on his clothes, never make an issue of it. You may remark, "All of us have accidents at times." Avoid making him feel guilty over his mistakes. Accompany your remarks with a sincere smile. This will help to relieve any tenseness the patient may feel over the accident.

18. Allow him to do whatever he thinks he can do for himself. Trying to give the patient help when he doesn't want it insults and discourages him. It often causes the patient to stop making any effort to help himself. If he can read, encourage him to read magazines or newspapers. If he can sign his name, suggest that he write it, rather than make a cross for his signature. If he can comb his hair or shave himself, let him do so. Everything he can do to take care of his grooming aids in building up his feelings of self-respect. Keep encouraging the patient to help himself in order to aid him in recovering his feelings of dignity and self-worth.

19. Avoid interrupting the patient when he is trying to tell you something. Should you try to say things for him, he will sense your impatience, tend to become discouraged, and not want to try to talk.

20. When the patient shows fatigue while trying to perform an activity, do not comment but offer to help him complete the task. If it is something which does not require completion (e.g., reading the newspaper), suggest a change of activity. Avoid saying to the patient, "You seem tired. Now let's do something else." Making such remarks to a patient—or to anyone, for that matter—is a negative suggestion and tends to make him feel more fatigued.

21. Avoid imposing your will upon the patient. Help him to make decisions for himself. Such attitudes as "Now you must do it this way" or "This is right because I say so" will only antagonize him. Strive to help him to do things because *he* wants to do them.

22. Avoid arguing with the patient. This is exhausting to him and makes him more angry or resentful.

23. Never scold, tease, or reprimand the patient in any way when he cannot perform a certain task. Such remarks are most discouraging and may cause him to lose all interest in making an effort.

24. Actually, an aphasic is usually more successful when performing an activity in which he shows intense interest. In such cases, never try to make him relax by such remarks as "Now relax; then you can say [this] or do [this]." Often the more intense he becomes, the better his progress will be.

© *Mary Coates Longerich 1955, 1958*

25. Should you get a letter from Aunt Sara telling how the crops have failed this year, or that Judge Brown's wife had a stroke last week, never discuss its contents with the patient. Unpleasant news of any kind might be upsetting to him. His concern now is *himself* and his own problems.
26. It is important to remember that no aphasic's problem is exactly like that of another. Therefore, avoid comparing him with anyone else.
27. Some form of occupational therapy may prove helpful for the patient. If he can actually contribute to the family income in any way, this will help to build his feeling of self-respect. For suggestions see L. Griswold, *Handicraft* (Outwest Printing, Colorado Springs, Colorado, 1945).
28. Avoid telling the patient "You'll soon be well." Such remarks are disillusioning to him. Be fair, honest, and direct in your dealings with him at all times. Avoid all discussions as to how long it will take him to recover. If the subject comes up, make some remark like, "It's true we have a job ahead of us, but we'll be doing all we can each day to move forward and reach our goals."
29. Direct the patient's attention to his improvement. Praise every bit of progress—even the tiniest improvement. Above all, be *sincere* in your comments. It is helpful for an aphasic to strive for specific goals—major goals, subgoals, and day-to-day goals. As these day-to-day goals are reached, praise him for his progress.
30. Never mention how the patient was before or after the injury, accident, or stroke. It doesn't help him; so avoid such discussions. Above all, refrain from discussing his speech disabilities with anyone in his presence.
31. Whenever you offer the patient an object, such as a comb, pronounce the word deliberately as you place it in his hand. It is important that he *hear* and *see* the word spoken at the split second the comb touches his hand.
32. When the patient indicates that he wants you to help him with a word, do whatever you can to assist him but make no mention of alphabet or spelling. The ability to spell is worked out automatically when the patient learns to write and say the word aloud as a unified process. For specific techniques see pages 22–26 of this manual, and Longerich and Bordeaux, *Aphasia Therapeutics,* pages 110–13 and 137–39 (The Macmillan Co., New York, 1954).
33. It will aid the patient greatly with his speech development if you assist him in recalling the names of his body parts. For example, as you help him wash his arm, say the word *arm* deliberately, *ah-r-m*. Exaggerate the lip and tongue movements as you say it. But make certain that you say *arm* as a whole word and not as a series of individual sounds. Utter the word at the split second that your hand touches the patient's arm. In a similar manner, help him with such words as *eye, ear, nose, throat,* etc. For example, in helping him with the word *eye* (*ah-ee*), open your mouth widely for the *ah*, then retract your lips similar to a smile for the *ee*. However, pronounce *eye* as a whole word, not in separate syllables. At the moment you start to utter *eye,* place your right index finger at the corner of your right eye. Encourage him to mirror your movements—that is, to place his left index finger at the corner of his left eye, as he tries to say *ah-ee*. In a similar manner, the patient may proceed to learn the names of other body parts. See page 11 of this manual. For suggestions and various detailed techniques, see pages 10–11 of this manual, and Longerich and Bordeaux, *Aphasia Therapeutics,* pages 109–56.
34. Frequent brief periods of practice on the various exercises (two to five times per day) are

© *Mary Coates Longerich 1955, 1958*

far more helpful to the aphasic than extended periods of practice. At first the patient may be able to work only a few moments (five or ten minutes) at a time. But, as he progresses, he most likely will be able to increase the length of practice periods. However, always discontinue practice when the patient feels tired. Try to close the session on a successful note; then immediately suggest some other activity which you think the patient will enjoy.

A question often asked by the family is, "Just how long will it take for my husband [or my wife] to develop speech?" The answer depends largely on the nature, extent, and severity of the injury. The most important point is that the patient get help with his aphasia problem as soon as possible after his accident, injury, or stroke.

Sometimes it is asked, "Will he be able to talk as well as he did before his accident or illness?" The answer is that rarely can the aphasic patient make a complete recovery. Frequently, however, he may seem to talk just as well as before the illness. There are certain of the more serious types of aphasia from which the patient can make only a partial speech recovery. Should you be able to help such an aphasic regain sufficient speech ability to make himself understood and his wants known, you can say to yourself, "This is a job well done!"

© *Mary Coates Longerich 1955, 1958*

part two

THE THERAPIST HELPS THE APHASIC

A. PLANNING APHASIA THERAPY
(For additional help, read the text, Longerich and Bordeaux, *Aphasia Therapeutics,* pages 97–156 [The Macmillan Co., New York, 1954].)

Because no one aphasic is exactly like another and no two aphasics' problems are the same, certainly it would not seem advisable to consider using exactly the same therapeutic procedures for any two aphasics. Instead, the need is to make a careful study of each patient's speech and language background and determine the areas of his loss. One aphasic may have a marked loss in speech, whereas another may have considerable residual speech but have difficulty in other realms.

To ascertain the patient's major therapeutic needs, of course a very thorough aphasia examination must be made. It is strongly recommended that this examination be administered by one who has had specialized training and experience in the field of aphasia. In case the patient lives in an isolated area and it is impossible to secure the professional help of an aphasia specialist, then the next best thing to do is to utilize the tests in the text, Longerich and Bordeaux, *Aphasia Therapeutics,* pages 65–87, in order to try to determine the patient's major areas of loss.

The important question to be answered by the aphasia tests is "What is this patient's greatest need?" For example, does he have a marked loss in the realm of understanding what he hears? An aphasia patient's hearing may be normal; his whole hearing mechanism may be intact. But because of brain damage he may not understand what he hears. Again, is the patient's major loss in the realm of eating? Is he markedly handicapped in recognizing what he sees, e.g., reading? Or, does he have a loss in the writing realm?

Of course, a patient may have one major problem, or he may have several. Selection of the area in which to begin therapy will depend not only upon the nature and the severity of the loss, but also upon the reactions of the patient; that is, in what area *he* feels is his greatest loss. For example, a patient's major handicap may be in the realm of reading, but he may also have some loss in the area of writing. Although reading is the more seriously affected area, the patient may have a strong urge to learn to sign his name. If this is his feeling, then therapy should begin with writing.

Some patients may be so severely handicapped that early therapy in the most serious realm will be of little help. In such case it will be necessary to start in an area in which the patient can make some progress.

Since it is evident that no two aphasics' problems are exactly the same, it would be next to impossible to plan a manual which could be followed step by step with every patient. Instead, only a general order of procedure can be recommended. And from these general suggestions a therapy program will need to be organized to fit each patient's needs.

For example, step 1, page 9, in the order of general procedure has to do with helping the patient to understand what he hears. If the aphasic has no major difficulty in understanding, but has a marked loss in ability to name concrete objects, then therapy should begin with step 2, page 9.

© Mary Coates Longerich 1955, 1958

Again, if a patient has four major problems—a difficulty in reading, a severe writing loss, a laborious and spasmodic utterance, as well as difficulty in masticating his food—then the first step of therapy would be to aid him in learning to chew and swallow his food. This would be indicated not only to help the patient with his eating, but also to aid him in his speech rehabilitation. Since the muscles of mastication are some of the same as those necessary for speech production, these muscles will necessarily have to be developed early in therapy. (See Preparing the Muscles for Speech, page 17.)

Of course, not all of the exercises and drills are suitable for every patient. One exercise may seem easy for one patient, while the same drill may seem difficult for another. Similarly, one patient may be able to do a drill in its entirety, whereas the same drill may have to have certain parts deleted to fit the needs of the next patient. So you as the therapist will have to appraise each exercise very carefully and decide whether it is suitable for the particular patient and whether any of the parts need to be omitted.

Of course, planning exercises and drills around the patient's hobbies, his interests, and his needs is very important for successful aphasia therapy. For a full discussion concerning the appraisal of the patient's capacities see the text, Longerich and Bordeaux, *Aphasia Therapeutics*, pages 61–88.

In order for an aphasic to be able to recover his speech, he will need at least some ability to understand the spoken word. Unfortunately, almost every aphasic has some difficulty, slight though it may be, in this auditory realm. Because people often tend to speak too rapidly to him, it is not unusual for the aphasic to misunderstand what he hears. It is important, therefore, to talk to the patient with well-articulated speech at a moderate rate of speed, approximately 125 to 140 words per minute. Day after day he needs to hear language spoken clearly and distinctly. In addition, of course, he needs systematic drills to help him in his speech and language development.

You will note that all the drills in Part Three are printed on perforated three-hole paper. With this format, the pages can be removed from the manual and inserted into an average-size loose-leaf notebook (obtainable at dime stores). It is suggested that you select the drill or drills which you wish to give to the patient at one particular session. Then let him insert them into his loose-leaf notebook if he can do so. In this way he will feel he is having at least a small part in compiling his handbook.

It is advisable that at each session the patient be given *only* the drill or drills which he will be using during that particular period. With this arrangement he will not have the opportunity of seeing other difficult exercises in the manual and becoming frustrated because he cannot do them. If he becomes discouraged, he may tend to withdraw into his shell and not want to make an effort.

One of the essentials of successful aphasia therapy is the patient's desire to help himself. Unless he is willing to exert every effort to move forward toward his goals, he cannot hope for much improvement.

The drills in Part Three have been divided into two sections: Drills for Receptive Aphasia, and Drills for Expressive Aphasia. The Receptive Aphasia section contains drills to aid the patient in understanding what he hears and in recognizing what he sees, e.g., the printed word. The Expressive Aphasia section comprises drills for helping the patient to communicate his ideas both in speech and in writing.

At the beginning of each set of drills in Part Three there are directions indicating how the therapist and patient are to proceed (see page 31). You will note that in some instances the phrase "to be read to the patient by the aphasia therapist" is added in parentheses. If just the word "directions" appears, this means that the patient is to read the instructions aloud if he

© *Mary Coates Longerich 1955, 1958*

can. If he is unable to do this, then the therapist and he are to read them aloud in unison. In case the patient still has difficulty, the therapist is to read the directions to him.

Following are suggested procedures for beginning aphasia therapy:

1. Talk to the patient about things within the level of his experience. For example, if the person is a carpenter, discuss the tools which he uses—his hammer, nails, and screws. If he is a pianist, then talk to him about the piano, the keyboard, pedals, etc. Or if the patient is a seamstress, discuss articles for sewing—needle, thread, thimble; how to use a sewing machine, how to make a dress, etc. Speak to the aphasic in well-articulated language. As suggested above, it will be necessary for the patient to hear good speech in order to be able to recover his speech.

2. If possible, devise some activity which will interest the patient, thereby stimulating him to language recall. For example, if the patient enjoyed playing a card game prior to his illness, plan a therapy program around this hobby. Some patients can relearn the names of the cards rather quickly by just playing the game a few times, whereas others will need much drill not only in recalling how the game is played but in relearning the names of the cards. Others, of course, may not benefit at all by this device. For some patients it is easier to learn the playing cards in this order: ace of clubs, ace of diamonds, ace of hearts, ace of spades; king of clubs, king of diamonds, king of hearts, king of spades; etc. Some will find it easier to say them in series, e.g., ace of clubs, two of clubs, three of clubs, etc.; whereas others will be able to recall the cards more quickly while playing the game. Again, adapt the procedure to the patient's needs. Usually this technique is more successful with aphasics who have some residual speech than with those who have little or no speech. Of course, the major purpose of such a device is to help the patient recall everyday speech, familiar expressions, etc. See Drill 85, page 201.

3. In case the patient has entirely lost the power of speech, begin the therapy program by asking him to point to certain objects in the room; for example, desk, chair, wall, lamp, floor, pencil, etc. Say the word in a modulated voice. As the patient points to the object, again name the object.

4. When he acquires skill in doing this, ask him to perform certain actions, e.g., "Turn on the light." Proceed similarly as you did for the individual words, making certain to repeat the request aloud as the patient performs the action. See Drill 1, page 31. Frequently the patient will begin to say a word or two of the directions with you. Encourage him to do so if he can. If the patient can just say a word or two, praise him for it.

5. Suggest to the patient: "I am going to point to various objects in the room. Name the object if you can. If you have difficulty, I will say the word. Then you try to say it with me." Later, the patient may begin to say the word which you have given. When this occurs, say: "Repeat what you said." This will aid the patient in gaining confidence in his own ability. If the patient has difficulty saying words with you, he may need concentrated drill on imitating lip and tongue movements. See Part Two, Section C, page 20.

6. Present to the patient action pictures such as those found in the large colored advertisements of *Life* and *Time* magazines and on the front covers of the *Saturday Evening Post*. Name various single objects in each picture and ask the patient to point to them.

7. Name the objects together with a descriptive phrase, for example, "The man with a red tie." "The girl who is crying." "The skater with the fur cap." Ask the patient to point to the various objects as they are named.

8. Name the single objects in the picture and suggest to the patient that he try to say them with you. Proceed as suggested in step 5 above.

© *Mary Coates Longerich 1955, 1958*

9. Have the patient try to name some of the objects in the picture. Assist him when he shows he needs help.
10. Use the *Longerich Aphasia Therapy Sets** in helping the patient to recall vocabulary. Talk about the objects on the picture cards in the same manner as you did the magazine pictures. Use five to ten pictures at a time. Place them in two or three rows in front of the patient and ask him to tell you anything about them that he can. If this is impossible for the patient, then name the objects in the pictures and suggest that he say them in unison with you when he is able to do so. (See procedure 5 above.) Usually it is better to work on five to ten pictures at a time, rather than two or three a day. Encourage the patient to talk about them in any way he can.

If the patient can read aloud, have him place five to ten pictures in one column and the corresponding cut-out labels in jumbled order in a second column; then try to match each word with the correct picture. As he matches the cut-out word with the picture, tell him to say the word aloud if he can. Next, he may place the same five to ten pictures in a column and try to name the objects aloud without looking at the cut-out words. If the patient cannot read aloud, then the cut-out word should be placed with each picture, so the patient will associate the printed word with the object. Later, he may practice naming the pictures without the words and reading the words without the pictures. For further drills in reading see procedures 14, 15, 16, 23, 24, 25, 26–31, 33–37, 39, 41–51, 54, and 63 and Drills 2–7, pages 33–43; also, Longerich and Bordeaux, *Aphasia Therapeutics,* pages 23–29, 42–54, 110–24.

11. Ask the patient questions which can be answered by *yes* or *no.* Suggestions for suitable questions may be found in Drills 8, 9, 10, and 11, pages 45–51.
12. Proceed similarly as in procedures 3 and 5 above in recalling the names of body parts. If the patient has difficulty, then he may first need practice naming the individual body parts. Have the patient sit beside you in front of a mirror. In this way he can watch your lips while you talk; then when he attempts to imitate what you have said, he can watch the movements of his own mouth.

To help him with the word *eye* (*ah-ee*), for instance, open your mouth widely for the *ah,* then retract your lips similar to a smile for the *ee.* However, pronounce *eye* as a whole word, not in separate syllables. At the moment you start to utter the word, place your left index finger at the corner of your left eye. Have him place his left index finger at the corner of his left eye and say the word *ah-ee* in unison with you.

Some emotionally disturbed patients become upset when asked to sit before a mirror, because it is difficult for them to face themselves as they are. In such case it is better to wait to use the mirror until after the patient has developed sufficient ego-strength to look at himself. Instead of his looking at the mirror, have him sit opposite you so he can watch your lips and tongue. Have him mirror your movements—that is, as the patient and you say the word *ah-ee* in unison, he is to place his left index finger at the corner of his left eye while you place your right index finger at the corner of your right eye.

The word *hand* may be taught in a similar manner. As you place your right hand on the patient's left hand, say *h-h* as a breath of air; *a-nd,* as one continuous word. Exaggerate the movement of lifting the tongue to the upper gum ridge for the *n* and *d.*

In helping him with the word *arm,* say the word very deliberately so he can watch the movements of your lips and tongue, e.g., *ah-r-m.* Be sure to say *arm* as a whole word and not just a succession of three separate sounds. Open your mouth widely for *ah;*

---

* The *Longerich Aphasia Therapy Sets* may be secured at cost ($1.75) by writing to the following address: Mary C. Longerich, Ph.D., 2007 Wilshire Boulevard, Los Angeles 57, California.

© Mary Coates Longerich 1955, 1958

square your lips as you say the sound of *r;* then press your lips together as you say *m.* Repeat the word several times as you lightly stroke his arm. It is important that he *hear* and *see* the word spoken at the moment that you place your hand on his arm.

Proceed in a similar fashion for recalling the names of other body parts such as ear, nose, face, leg, knee, foot, toe, etc. Next, try naming the body parts in series. For example, pointing to each body part the split second you name it, say very slowly in rhythm: "Eye, ear, nose, and throat." Exaggerate lip and tongue movements as you say the words in a modulated voice. Suggest to the patient, "Try to say the words with me." In case the patient has difficulty emulating certain sounds, see Part Two, Section C and E. Following is a suggested list of body parts, clothing, food, etc., which may be learned in series in a similar manner as described for "eye, ear, nose, and throat" above.

BODY PARTS
- I. eye
  - ear
  - nose
  - throat
- II. arm
  - hand
  - thumb
  - finger
- III. leg
  - foot
  - toe
  - heel
- IV. eyebrow
  - eyelash
  - mouth
- V. elbow
  - wrist
  - knee
  - ankle
- VI. hair
  - cheek
  - lip
  - teeth
- VII. head
  - shoulder
  - neck
  - hip
- VIII. chin
  - chest
  - heart
  - back

CLOTHING
- I. hat
  - coat
  - shirt
  - trousers
- II. shoes
  - socks
  - tie
  - belt
- III. pajamas
  - bathrobe
  - slippers
- IV. sweater
  - shorts
  - shoelaces
  - undershirt

FURNISHINGS
- I. wall
  - door
  - window
  - floor
- II. couch
  - desk
  - chair
  - lamp
- III. bed
  - dresser
  - mirror
  - rug
- IV. bathtub
  - washbowl
  - shower
  - towel
- V. sink
  - stove
  - table
  - stool
- VI. drapes
  - picture
  - plant
  - fireplace

FOOD
- I. bread
  - butter
  - jam
  - milk
- II. steak
  - potatoes
  - gravy
  - beans
- III. apples
  - oranges
  - pears
  - grapes
- IV. ham
  - eggs
  - toast
  - coffee
- V. soup
  - meat
  - salad
  - dessert

MISCELLANEOUS
- I. car
  - hood
  - tire
  - bumper
- II. radio
  - clock
  - camera
  - television
- III. paper
  - pencil
  - pen
  - ink

© Mary Coates Longerich 1955, 1958

To facilitate the naming of clothing, furnishings, food, etc., it is recommended that the actual articles in the patient's everyday environment be used when it is convenient. For example, in learning to say the word *door,* it is helpful to pronounce the word *door* at the split second you point to it. In addition to using the actual objects for the learning of such a word as *door,* it is also helpful to use a picture of it. Again, at the very moment that you point to the door in the picture, say *door.* See procedure 15, page 12; Drill 69, page 169; also Longerich and Bordeaux, *Aphasia Therapeutics,* pages 113–20.

13. When the patient is able to repeat single words, he may be given short phrases such as: "red book," "big dog," "white house," etc. Then short conversational sentences may be used such as:

    a. Good morning.
    b. How are you?
    c. Hello.
    d. Thank you.
    e. Pardon me.
    f. Good night.
    g. Come here.

    The length of phrases and sentences may be gradually increased, e.g., "Please pass me the salt." "Open the door." See Drill 85, page 201.

    Suggest to the patient that he observe very carefully the movements of your lips and your tongue. "Notice what I do at the beginning of the word—what I do with my lips. Watch each syllable, and look at the end of each word. Observe very carefully as I pronounce each word in the sentence."

14. To aid the patient in recalling the names of objects and in reading, it is suggested that work begin on writing during the very first days of therapy. At this point it should be mentioned that, while the patient learns to speak and write a word as a unified process, no mention of spelling need be made. This problem is automatically resolved as the patient learns to integrate the sound with the written word. For specific writing techniques, see Part Two, Section D, and Longerich and Bordeaux, *Aphasia Therapeutics,* pages 112–17. In addition, see Drills 70–84, pages 171–99.

15. To help the patient achieve further speech, use object-pictures in Courtis and Watters' *Illustrated Golden Dictionary* (Simon and Shuster, Inc., New York, 1951). Cut out and place a picture, e.g., *hen,* on a sheet of notebook paper and write or print the name of the object below it. Proceed similarly as explained in procedures 5–9 above.

16. Place five to ten object-pictures on a page. Arrange the names of the objects in a jumbled word list and have the patient associate each word with its object. See Drills 2–4, pages 33–37, and Drill 7, page 43.

17. You may ask the patient to count with you; for example, 1-2-3-4-5. Try to say the words meaningfully and in a rhythmical pattern, emphasizing the word *five.* Usually it helps to count objects or to point to numerical figures as you practice this. For example, you may number the digits on one hand. Point to the thumb when you say *one,* to the index finger as you say *two,* and so on up to *five.* Similarly, count to 10; 20; 30; etc.

    With some patients it is helpful to write the numerical figures 1 to 5 on paper and ask the patient to say the words with you as you point to each number on the paper. As soon as he can count to five, then write the numbers 1 to 10 and proceed in a similar fashion. Usually, it is easier to learn numbers in groups of five.

© Mary Coates Longerich 1955, 1958

18. Repeat a series of numbers and have the patient respond. For example:

    7 — 9
    8 — 11
    4 — 7 — 2
    8 — 6 — 9
    2 — 4 — 7 — 5
    8 — 2 — 3 — 9
    6 — 1 — 4 — 7
    6 — 3 — 2 — 8 — 9
    8 — 1 — 4 — 6 — 5

    See Drill 15, page 59.

19. Patients may be asked to say the days of the week in unison with you. Proceed in a similar manner as discussed in step 12 above. Often it helps to say the days of the week somewhat in rhythm, for this seems to aid many patients in going from one word to the next. Also, months of the year may be practiced in a similar fashion.

20. Say to the patient:

    "Today is _____."
    "Yesterday was _____."
    "Tomorrow is _____."

21. Perform actions, e.g., knocking on the table. Ask the patient to tell you what you are doing. See Drill 86, page 203.

22. Present pictures (as described in procedure 6 above) and ask the patient to name the objects and tell one thing about them. For example: dog-runs; boy-laughs; father-eats; etc.

23. Say the first part of a sentence and let the patient tell the last word. See Drill 87, page 205; also, Longerich and Bordeaux, *Aphasia Therapeutics,* page 119.

24. Ask the patient to find a particular word each time it appears in a given group of words. See Drills 19–23, pages 67–75.

25. Give the patient a list of eight or ten words which contain four or five words in a certain category, e.g., foods. Have him check all of the words in that category. See Drills 16–18, pages 61–65.

26. Give the patient a list of three to five words. Read aloud one of the words in the group and have him point to it. See Drill 19, page 67.

27. Write certain sentences, e.g., "The dog runs," and suggest to the patient that he read them aloud with you. After you have read the sentences several times in unison, suggest to the patient that he may be able to read some of the words alone. Often the patient will find he can read a word within a sentence by first looking at the entire sentence. Or, he may be able to read the final word of a phrase or sentence, if you read to him the first part of it. Other sentences which may be used are:

    a. I eat bacon and _____.   (eggs)
    b. I wash my _____.   (hands)
    c. A bird _____.   (sings)
    d. We go to _____.   (church)
    e. I shave with my _____.   (razor)
    f. I wind my _____.   (watch)
    g. I saw a ball _____.   (game)
    h. My name is _____.

© Mary Coates Longerich 1955, 1958

i. I live in _____(city)_____.

j. My husband's (or wife's) name is _____.

See Drill 87, page 205.

28. Ask the patient to sing with you a familiar song (preferably one he knew in his adolescence). Avoid using nursery rhymes, for they seem too childish to an adult patient. First sing the song with the patient, having him watch your lip movements and joining with you whenever he can. Next, write the words of the song and ask him to sing the words with you as you both point to them on the paper. Make no issue over the patient's omitting words in the song as you sing together. The important thing is for you to "keep going" with the song. Sing the words deliberately but with rhythm, making certain that both you and the patient point to each word the moment it is sung. As soon as the patient is singing most of the words of the song with you, stop singing at various points which seem easiest for him and let him continue for a word or two or perhaps a few short phrases on his own. When he begins to show signs of faltering, start immediately singing in unison with him to help him to "carry on." Make no correction if the patient mispronounces a word, but commend him for the parts he can say. Practice until the patient can sing the song alone. Or, if he grows weary of this song, select another very familiar one and proceed in a similar way. When he can sing the song without your help, suggest that he say the words in rhythmical speech (but not singing it). As soon as he can do this, then you may start working on the individual words. At this point, he may be able to find individual words or phrases in the song that he can read aloud. If he cannot do this, then you name individual words and have the patient point to the written word and repeat it after you. Later he may be able to read the words without your help.

29. Read aloud a short anecdote such as may be found in the *Reader's Digest* or *Coronet*. Make certain that the material is within the scope of the patient's experience. Proceed similarly as with the song. First read the anecdote aloud. Suggest that both you and the patient point to each word so he may follow the words as you read them. Tell the patient to join in reading with you whenever he can do so. As soon as he is reading most of the anecdote in unison with you, stop reading at various points and let the patient carry on when he can. But if he begins to hesitate, again start reading with him so he may maintain the rhythm of easy-flowing speech. Sometimes it is surprising how soon a patient can join in and actually read aloud several words.

30. Give the patient a phrase, then ask him to select one word among a group of three words that means the same as the phrase. See Drill 24, pages 77–78.

31. To help the patient increase his vocabulary, select a slightly more difficult anecdote. However, the material must not be too involved for the patient, for in such case he would feel overwhelmed and might tend to draw within his shell and say nothing. As the patient becomes able to join in the reading of various words and phrases, gradually increase the rate of reading until you have reached a moderate speed (approximately 125 to 140 words per minute).

32. Practice antonyms. Give the patient a word and ask him to tell you its opposite. See Drill 88, page 207; and Longerich and Bordeaux, *Aphasia Therapeutics,* page 123.

33. Point to a word and ask the patient to point to its antonym and say it aloud, if he can. See Drill 25, page 79, and Drill 88, page 207.

34. Have the patient look at a group of four to six words, and select the words that rhyme. See Drills 26 and 27, pages 81–82.

© *Mary Coates Longerich 1955, 1958*

35. Give the patient a word such as *hat* and ask him to tell you some words rhyming with *hat* (for example: *bat, cat*). Other words to be used are *man* (*pan, can, ran*); *pin* (*tin, win, kin*); *pen* (*ten, den, hen*). See Drill 89, page 209.
36. Give the patient some words such as *hat* and ask him to write three or four words that rhyme with it. See Drills 89–92, pages 209–15.
37. Ask the patient to match words that rhyme. See Drills 26 and 27, pages 81–83.
38. Ask the patient to give you a word in a certain category that rhymes with another word, e.g., "Name a food that rhymes with *lake*." See Drill 90, page 211.
39. Have the patient read lists of words which belong to particular sound families. See Drill 93, page 217.
40. Present a situational picture to the patient and ask him to tell you one thing about it. For example, a mother feeding her baby, a man mowing the lawn. See procedure 7 above.
41. Ask the patient to read word groups that look similar. See Drills 94–97, pages 219–25.
42. Have the patient find the little words in a longer word. See Drills 28–32, pages 85–93.
43. The patient may be asked to underline the words in a group of sentences which contain a certain sound. See Drills 34–37, pages 97–103.
44. Have the patient match words in one column that correspond in meaning to the words or phrases of another column. See Drills 38–44, pages 105–17.
45. Select four or five simple headlines from the newspaper and paste them on a page of the patient's notebook paper. Proceed similarly as in procedure 23 above.
46. Select a short human-interest story from the newspaper. Usually a story accompanied by a picture helps to motivate the patient's reading. Proceed with the reading of the news article as described in step 23 above.
47. As the patient improves in his reading ability, gradually longer and more difficult anecdotes from magazines and news articles from the paper may be given to him. Follow the procedure as described in step 23 above. At first, it will be necessary for you to read the material in unison with the patient before he tries to do it alone. However, as soon as he feels he can read it at sight, encourage him to do so by himself.
48. Present incomplete sentences to the patient and have him supply the suitable words. See Drills 45–65, pages 119–59.
49. Give the patient a list of words or short phrases and have him arrange them into a sentence. If he has difficulty, place each word on a slip of paper, then have him arrange the words in order. See Drills 66–68, pages 161–65.
50. Have the patient write the complete form of a word containing a contraction, e.g., *I'm—I am*. See Drill 98, page 227.
51. Have the patient read questions and write the answer *yes* or *no*. See Drills 99–100, pages 229–31.
52. Give the patient a certain word and ask him to name all of the things of which this word reminds him. It is important to use stimulus words within the experience and interest of the patient.
53. Read each of these sentences to the patient and ask him, "Tell me what I am talking about in each sentence."
    a. Bill's horse won the race today.
    b. Jane is coming home today.
    c. Bob has a new Jaguar car.
    d. The Smiths are going to Europe.

© *Mary Coates Longerich 1955, 1958*

54. Have the patient read an anecdote (see procedure 23 above); then ask him simple questions about the anecdote. The patient may respond with only a word or two; he may make his answer by saying or pointing to just one word; and/or he may write the answers. See Drills 101–104, pages 233–39.
55. Give the patient a direction and ask him to tell what you said, but not necessarily with the same words you used. For example:
    a. Tell the maid to have dinner at six o'clock.
    b. Go to the store and get a pound of butter and a loaf of bread.
    c. Tell John to wash the car Saturday afternoon.

    As the patient's abilities develop, materials of increasing length and difficulty may be used.
56. Read short paragraphs to the patient and ask him to tell what each is about.
57. Read a news article to the patient and ask him to tell the main idea.
58. Ask the patient to listen to a radio newscast or a telecast and tell about it.
59. Ask the patient to describe the following objects: apple, dog, barn, house, etc. It is very important to use words involving the special interests of the patient.
60. Ask the patient how to perform certain tasks. Again select those things the individual will enjoy doing. For example:
    a. How to light a cigarette.
    b. How to wash a car.
    c. How to swim.
    d. How to bake a cake.

    See Drill 105, page 241.
61. Ask the patient questions regarding points of the compass, e.g., "What direction would you have to face so that your right arm would be toward the west?" See Drill 106, page 243.
62. Read an absurd statement to the patient and ask him to tell you what is foolish or odd about the idea. Similarly, let the patient read the statement and tell what is unusual about it. For example:
    a. We keep our milk in the stove.
    b. The rooster chased the swan across the lake.
    c. We use ice to heat our house.
    d. The sun shines at night.
    e. I sleep while I eat my lunch.

    For additional sentences see Drills 107–108, pages 245–47.
63. Ask the patient to read questions such as "Which can you hear?" (chair, radio, rug) and encircle the correct answer. See Drill 110, page 251.
64. Give the patient questions requiring reasoning. See Drill 109, page 249.
65. Have the patient show how certain pairs of words are alike, e.g., *pen* and *pencil*. See Drills 111–115, pages 253–61.
66. Ask the patient questions regarding the value of money. See Drill 116, pages 263–64.
67. Give the patient a group of numbers in sequence. Ask him to supply the next two numbers that would follow. See Drill 117, page 265.
68. Give the patient a paragraph containing 10 to 15 directions which can be performed with pencil and paper. See Drills 118–119, pages 267–69.

© *Mary Coates Longerich 1955, 1958*

THE THERAPIST HELPS THE APHASIC · 17

69. Give the patient incomplete sentences pertaining to general information and have him supply the needed words. See Drills 120–121, pages 271–73.
70. Give the patient a list of adverbs and ask him to place each word in the column under the appropriate heading: *how, when,* or *where.* See Drill 123, page 277.
71. Ask the patient to read a list of words which refer to things he can either "do" or "smell." Have him place each word under the appropriate category. See Drill 122, page 275.

B. PREPARING THE MUSCLES FOR SPEECH

If the patient has marked difficulty in masticating his food, he probably will have trouble with articulation also. Since many of the muscles used for chewing, sucking, and swallowing are used also for speech, a patient will require a certain facility in utilizing this apparatus in order to make speech understandable. Hence, a patient's learning to masticate his food is one of the first steps toward his speech recovery. Following are exercises you may use to help the patient in the rehabilitation of these muscles:

I. Yawning Exercise

Yawning is one of the best exercises for training of the soft palate. Whenever the patient "accidentally" yawns, encourage him to yawn again.

II. Blowing Exercises

A. Blow a feather across the table.
B. Blow out a match.
C. Blow out or bend the flame of a very small candle; then a larger one.
D. Blow a small whistle. If the patient has difficulty holding it with his lips, suggest that he hold on to it with his teeth. If he has difficulty closing his teeth over the whistle, you may aid him in the following way:
   1. Sit facing the patient and hold the whistle with your left thumb and index finger.
   2. With the middle finger of your left hand, hold the patient's upper lip over the whistle.
   3. Place the palm of your right hand on the patient's chin; move the chin upward until the patient's lower lip touches the whistle.
   4. Then say to the patient, "Bite the whistle; now blow!"
   5. In case the patient has difficulty blowing, have him first practice the exercise of emitting a sigh. Demonstrate the exercise by first doing it yourself. Place your hand at your diaphragm, just below the sternum (at the waist). As you inhale air, move your hand outward.* Then as you exhale, i.e., make the sigh, move your hand inward. Placing your hand on your abdomen, just below the sternum, will help the patient visualize the inward and outward movements during the process of inhalation and exhalation. Of course, the shoulders should remain steady during the exercise. Give two or three demonstrations of sighing; then ask the patient to do it. Place your hand lightly at the patient's diaphragm, i.e., just below the sternum (at the waist). Say to him, "Move your waist outward

---

*It is understood that during the process of inhalation the diaphragm moves downward as the waist moves outward. Similarly, during exhalation the diaphragm moves upward as the waist moves inward. Usually it is better to omit such an explanation to an aphasic, for it probably would be too involved for him to understand.

© *Mary Coates Longerich 1955, 1958*

as you inhale; then relax and let your waist move inward as you make the sigh. Be sure to keep your shoulders steady during the exercise."

    E. Blow up a small sack; then a larger one.

    F. Blow up a small balloon; then a larger one.

III. Lip Exercises

    A. Pucker the lips as for a kiss.

    B. Smile broadly, then pucker the lips as for a kiss.
Alternate the two movements three or four times.

IV. Jaw Exercise

To aid the patient in relearning of jaw movements, place the palm of your right hand on the chin of the patient and help him to open and close his jaw *very slowly*. Suggest to the patient, "Now let the jaw relax." Then move the jaw slowly up and down, quietly saying, "up-down; up-down." As soon as he can move his jaw with your help, coax him to try it alone.

V. Tongue Exercises

    A. Ask the patient to protrude his tongue. If he has difficulty doing this, suggest that he place his own hand on his chin and move it downward. Usually moving of the lower jaw downward will aid in the protruding of the tongue. In case the patient cannot use his own hand to move his lower jaw, ask if he would like you to help him. Proceed in opening his mouth as described in the Jaw Exercise (IV) above. Continue working on this exercise four or five times a day, until the patient can protrude his tongue at least as far forward as the lower lip.

    B. As soon as the patient can move his tongue forward and touch the lower lip, proceed with this next exercise. Take a piece of paper toweling and fold it to the shape of a rectangle, 1 inch x 2 inches. Make certain you have several thicknesses of paper in the rectangle. Take hold of the patient's tongue by placing one end of the toweling below the tongue and the other end above it. Suggest to the patient, "Just let your tongue relax." Then move the tongue slowly up and down four or five times. Let the patient rest a few moments. Again take hold of the tongue as described above and move the tongue from left to right four or five times. When the tongue begins to move more easily, suggest to the patient, "You help me move your tongue." In this way you may teach him to move his tongue himself.

    C. As soon as he can move his tongue without your help (this may take several weeks or even months), suggest that he move his tongue up and down slowly to the count of six; then right and left to the count of six.

    D. Put applesauce on the patient's tongue. If he has difficulty moving the food about in his mouth, insert a tongue depressor to help him in the process.

    E. Put preserves or jam on the patient's lower lip. Encourage him to lick it off.

    F. Place some peanut butter on the roof of his mouth, just behind the upper front teeth. Encourage him to lick it off. Hold the chin down so he will not tend to use the jaw muscles to reach for the peanut butter.

    G. Put a piece of sugar cookie or graham cracker

        1. between the patient's lower lip and his lower teeth.

        2. in the corner of the patient's mouth.

© Mary Coates Longerich 1955, 1958

3. in the cheek outside the teeth.*

Say to him, "Try to get the cookie." After he can do these exercises, you may use small pieces of meat. You will find that these will retain their shape for a longer period of time.

H. Encourage the patient to "wipe the ice cream" off his mouth by licking his upper lip, his lower lip, the corners of his mouth, etc.

VI. Sucking Exercises

Teaching the patient to suck through a tube will facilitate his taking of liquids, and also will help to stop drooling. Moreover, it will aid markedly in the development of lip movements and breathing habits necessary for speech.

Secure a 6-inch piece of surgical rubber tubing of about 1/4-inch diameter. The walls of the tube should be thick and durable so as to open again after being bitten. Wash the tube thoroughly; otherwise the patient may get a "rubber taste" when he uses it. Dip one end into a liquid such as soup, meat broth, or fruit juice. Then place your right index finger (if you are right-handed) on the other end of the tube. Fill 2 or 3 inches of the tube with the liquid. Place your left thumb on his lower lip, helping him to hold his lips over the end of the tube. Hold the tube horizontally and allow the liquid to flow into his mouth. Practice this exercise two or three times per day.†

Continue these procedures for about a month or six weeks, or until the patient is able to hold the tube with his lips and can let the liquid flow into his mouth.

Next, begin holding the tube at a slight angle below the horizontal position, and say, "See if you can get the soup. Put your lips around the tube; run your tongue around and around on the inside edge of the tube." As you give these suggestions, raise the tube horizontally for a few seconds, then lower it again, so that he will begin to *want* to move his tongue around in the hole and then pull it out. Diligent work on this exercise should aid in the development of a slight sucking movement. Lower the tube a little bit each week, proceeding in a similar manner as described above.

As soon as the patient has learned to use the surgical tubing for sucking, let him use a plastic tube. Secure a cup with a plastic cover.‡ Bore a small hole in the center of the lid and insert a 3-inch length of plastic tubing. Again assist the patient by placing your right thumb (if you are right-handed) on his upper lip, helping him to hold his lips over the end of the tube. Then put the remaining part of your right hand beneath his chin in order to give his face the needed support. Hold the cup with your left hand. As soon as he has learned to suck through this plastic tube, use a 4-inch tube; later, a 5-inch tube, etc. Next, he may be given a hard-plastic commercial tube; finally, a regular waxed straw from a soda fountain.

In order to remind the patient to use his straw when drinking liquids, place the straw on the table with his silverware.

VII. Chewing and Swallowing Exercises

A. Place a small piece of bubble gum or ordinary gum in the patient's mouth. Demonstrate the chewing motions needed to move the gum around in his

---

* Westlake, Harold: A System for Developing Speech," *The Crippled Child*, 24:12-13, 1951.
† Palmer, Martin F.: "Studies in Clinical Techniques," *J. Speech Disorders*, 12:416-18, 1947.
‡ Levinson, Helen J.: "A Parent Training Program for a Cerebral Palsy Unit," *J. Speech & Hearing Disorders*, 19:254-55, 1954.

© *Mary Coates Longerich 1955, 1958*

mouth. Let him have the gum for only a few seconds (not more than 30 seconds); then retrieve it. Gradually increase the length of time for him to have the gum in his mouth. Practice this exercise at least once a day for a period of four to six weeks. As the patient develops ability in chewing, he will find that in order to enjoy his gum he must learn to swallow the saliva.* Another means of teaching the patient to swallow saliva, thereby alleviating the drooling problem, is to suggest to him that he hold his mouth shut with his hand frequently during the day.

B. If he has difficulty learning to chew gum, let him practice chewing a gumdrop. Tie a piece of string to the gumdrop. Place it in his mouth, preferably between his teeth. Encourage him to move it around in his mouth as in chewing. As soon as he has chewed the gumdrop for a few seconds (not more than 30 or 40 seconds), remove the gumdrop from his mouth by the string. Then repeat the process. This exercise should be practiced at a given hour at least once a day.

As soon as the patient has developed skill in chewing, insert the gumdrop in his mouth without the string. Start counting the chewing motions and encourage him to swallow. For example, "One-two-three-four, swallow; one-two-three-four, swallow."

C. Place dry, sliced bread on the window sill or in the oven until it is quite hard. Give him a piece of this bread at each meal. Raw turnip or carrot sticks also are excellent foods for helping him to learn to chew and swallow. (Let it be emphasized that these foods and the liquids mentioned in this manual are *not* recommended as diet for the patient. They are merely suggested foods for the exercises of sucking, chewing, and swallowing—movements which are vital for his speech development. Consult your physician regarding foods which he should eat.)

As you proceed with these exercises, try to instill in him the courage and the determination to succeed. Even though he finds these exercises tedious, help him to understand that he must learn to use his speech musculature adequately in order to be able to imitate the words he *sees* and *hears*.

C. IMITATING LIP AND TONGUE MOVEMENTS
(See Longerich and Bordeaux, *Aphasia Therapeutics,* pages 139–40.)

If the patient has difficulty in repeating words which he hears, he may need training not only in the use of his speech musculature (see Section B), but he may require help in other realms also. For example, he may need auditory drills to aid him in understanding what is said to him (see Drills 1, 9, 15, and 19, pages 31, 47, 59, and 67, respectively). In addition, he may need exercises to teach him how to imitate the actual lip and tongue movements of the words which he sees and hears. The following exercises are suggested to develop the ability to imitate lip and tongue movements:

I. The patient and therapist are seated facing a mirror (at least 2 feet square). The therapist performs the tongue exercise; then the patient tries to execute the movements which he has observed. In case the mirror proves emotionally upsetting to the patient, have him sit opposite you.

---
* Palmer, Martin F.; *op. cit.,* p. 417.

© *Mary Coates Longerich 1955, 1958*

For example:
- A. Retract lips.
- B. Purse lips.
- C. Retract lips; purse lips.
- D. Purse lips; retract lips; purse lips.
- E. Place the tongue tip at the top of the upper lip, then close the mouth. Next place the tongue at a point just below the lower lip, i.e., just above the chin. Close the mouth. It is important that the lips be closed for a second or two between each tongue movement. As soon as the therapist has performed the up-and-down movements of the tongue, the patient is asked to imitate the action. All tongue movements are performed slowly.
- F. Next, the therapist moves his own tongue to the right corner of his mouth, then to the left. Following this procedure, the patient is requested to do the same. In case the patient finds it too frustrating to sit in front of the mirror, he should sit opposite you and imitate what he *sees* you do. For example, if you move your tongue to the right, then he moves his tongue to his left, etc.
- G. As soon as the patient can do the two tongue exercises above, they may be combined in various ways.
    1. Left, right
    2. Right, up
    3. Down, left
    4. Down, up, right
    5. Up, left, down
    6. Right, down, up
    7. Up, down, right, left
    8. Up, right, up, left
    9. Up, down, right, down
    10. Right, left, up, down
    11. Left, right, up, left
    12. Up, down, up, right, left
    13. Left, right, up, down, right

    Similarly, other combinations of the above tongue movements may be used. At the first it is better to do only three or four sets of exercises at a practice period. Later, as the patient's skills develop, the number of exercises may be gradually increased. The important thing to keep in mind is that the period of practice should end on a successful note.

II. Next, tongue exercises may be combined with simple words. For example:
- A. Up, down, "I."
- B. Right, left, "O."
- C. Up, left, "arm." (Place your right hand on your left arm at the split second you say "arm.")
- D. Right, up, "ear." (Place your right index finger on your right ear at the moment you say "ear.")
- E. Up, down, right, "nose." (Place your finger on your nose while you say "nose.")

See procedure 12, page 10.

© Mary Coates Longerich 1955, 1958

D. WRITING

(For additional helps, read the text, Longerich and Bordeaux, *Aphasia Therapeutics,* pages 23–29, 42–44, 54, and 110–24; and Gardner, Warren. *Left-Handed Writing* [Interstate Press, Danville, Illinois, 1945].)

As mentioned before (Part Two, Section A, procedure 14, page 3), drills in writing should begin very early in aphasia therapy, preferably during the first or second week. Because the large percentage of aphasics have a right-sided paralysis (i.e., right hemiplegia), the right hand frequently is paralyzed to the extent that it cannot be used for major skills (e.g., eating, shaving, writing, etc.). Therefore, the left hand necessarily has to be employed for the writing process. With some aphasics, neither of the patient's hands may be paralyzed. If such be the case, frequently it is wise for the aphasic to change hands for his major skills, e.g., use his left hand instead of his right. But the decision for such a change *must* come from the physician-in-charge. *Never* should a therapist recommend to the patient a shift in handedness, for only the physician understands fully the neurological and physiological implications. (For a discussion of the neurological and physiological aspects of the aphasic, see the text, Longerich and Bordeaux, *Aphasia Therapeutics,* pages 3–14, 23, 27, 30–35, 37–38, 44–46, 52, 54–55, and 57.)

Training in writing should begin just as soon as the patient is able to emulate the therapist in saying such words as *O* and *I*. Have the patient sit in front of a mirror; then you stand behind him so he can watch your lip, tongue, and hand movements in the mirror. Take the patient's hand and help him write and say the word *O* in the air. At the moment that you make the downstroke of the letter *O,* say *O*. Next, ask the patient to say and write the word with you as the two of you face the mirror. Again, be sure to say and write the word *O* as a *unified* procedure. If the patient is greatly disturbed by watching himself in the mirror, you need not use the mirror. Sit beside the patient and perform the exercise as described above.

As soon as the patient has attained skill in saying and writing the word *O* in the air, suggest that he say it and trace it. First write the letter *O* (approximately 3 to 4 inches high) on a piece of paper. With your index finger say and trace the word *O* several times. Then, holding the patient's writing hand, help him to trace and write it until he seems to do it with assurance. Next, have the patient write and say the word alone, without looking at the model he has traced. For the patient's writing it is preferable to use paper with lines at least ⅜ inch apart. At first the *O* should be at least ½ inch in height. (See Drill 70, page 171.) Later, when the patient attains more skill, smaller letters may be made.

Have the patient practice saying and writing *O* until he can do it with comparative ease; then start with the word *I* and proceed in a similar manner as for *O*. (See Drill 71, page 173.) In the case of *I,* again the word is uttered just as you begin to make the downstroke of the letter.

Next, a simple word such as *no* may be used. For example, in writing the word before the mirror, say the word on the downstroke of each sound, e.g., utter the sound of *n* (not the letter *ĕn*!) at the moment the downstroke of *n* is made. Then say *o* as you make the downstroke of the letter *o*. Note that the word is written and said as a unified process, i.e., in slow motion as a continuous succession of sounds, *nnn-o-o-o*. See Drill 72, page 175.

Next, ask the patient to say and write the word without looking at the model he has traced. It is most important that the patient *not* copy the word, but write it entirely from memory. If he has trouble doing this, then he needs to return to the large word he traced, and practice saying and simultaneously tracing it with his index finger.

One of the questions frequently asked about writing therapy by the new aphasia therapist is: "Because the majority of aphasics have a right-sided paralysis (i.e., right hemiplegia) and of necessity have to use the left hand for writing, wouldn't it be an easier and faster process for

© *Mary Coates Longerich 1955, 1958*

them to learn to print rather than to write?" During the past quarter of a century's experience in the field of speech pathology, the author has not found this to be the case. Instead, printing seems to be the long way out. Since in printing, the patient usually does not connect his letters as he does in writing, he is inclined to think of the letters as separate units rather than as a continuous succession of sounds. Consequently, he is prone to spell the word aloud as he prints, instead of saying the word in "slow motion." When he spells the word, this means he goes through an added step in learning, thus prolonging the therapy process. For example, in working on the word *cat,* he would have to learn (1) to say it; (2) to spell it; and (3) to print it. Whereas, if he said and wrote the word as a unified process, it would involve fewer learning procedures. For this reason, it is strongly recommended that the patient write his words rather than print them.

In some instances, of course, it may be next to impossible for the aphasic to learn to write. In such case, it is necessary to have him try to learn to print.

Some aphasics who print have difficulty in making such letters as *h* in *hat, r* in *rug, k* in *back, l* in *leg,* and *t* in *top.* Frequently they write individual letters backwards, e.g., и in *no* rather than *n.* Some aphasics start at the right and move to the left as they print the *n,* rather than moving from left to right. This problem is called mirror writing. In case your patient has this difficulty, tell him to begin his letter at the extreme upper left-hand side of the page and move from left to right. Demonstrate this to him if necessary.

Make certain to use whole words (not single letters) when demonstrating to a patient how to say or print a word. Show him how to print the word from left to right, using the downward stroke. For example:

no   ball   pea

For additional examples and suggestions for printing, see the text, Longerich and Bordeaux, *Aphasia Therapeutics,* pages 111–12.

To help the patient to utter each sound on the downstroke of the letter, it is often helpful to prepare a writing sheet for the patient. Write (or print, if necessary) the word in cursive letters (⅜ to ½ inch high) three or four times at the top of the page. Draw double lines vertically between the words; also, a single vertical line down the page between each sound, e.g., *n* and *o.* Tell the patient it is very important to write (or print) and say the word on the downstroke, and to wait to start the next sound until *after* he has crossed the vertical line. This is necessary to facilitate associating the written letter with the corresponding sound.

Although the model words are written at the top of the page, the patient does *not* copy them. He places a paper or "hide sheet" over what has been written, and proceeds to write and say the word. He should not be allowed to erase or cross out a letter or word. Instead, he should cover it with his hide sheet and try again to say and write the word.

Note that *no mention of the alphabet or of spelling ever need be made* to the patient. By learning to integrate the sound with the writing, much of the labor of spelling can be eliminated. This saves hours of work in retraining.

After teaching the aphasic to write and say *no,* the person may be given such words as *arm, ear, nose,* etc. (See Drills 73–75, pages 177–81.) In saying and writing (or printing) the word *arm,* pronounce *ah* on the downstroke of the letter *a;* say *r* as in the word *her* (not *R* as in R.S.V.P.) on the downstroke of the letter *r;* and *m* as in *me* on the downward stroke of the letter *m.* Make certain that the word *arm* is said as a continuous succession of sounds, e.g., *ah-rr-mm.*

In the word *ear,* which has a silent letter in the middle of the word, pronounce the *e* on the

© Mary Coates Longerich 1955, 1958

downstroke of the *e;* say nothing while writing the letter *a;* then utter *r* as in *her* as you write the letter *r*. Similarly, with the word *nose,* the *n, o,* and *s* are said and written on the downstroke of each respective sound; then the *e* is written with no utterance of sound because it is a silent letter.

Frequently questions arise as to how certain words should be said during the writing process, for example, such words as *ball, pea,* and *pot*. In saying and writing (or printing) the word *ball,* the word is said aloud as a continuous succession of sounds. The sound of *b* is pronounced *buh* (not *bee,* as the second letter of the alphabet); the sound *a* in *ball* is pronounced *aw* (as in *law*), not as the letter *a* in the word *ate;* the first *l* is pronounced like *l* in the word *hill,* not like the letter *el* in the abbreviation L.S.U. (Louisiana State University). Note that this first sound of *l* may be continued through the writing of the final *l;* or the final *l* may be written in silence.

In saying and writing or printing the word *pea,* the *p* is whispered (*not* said aloud) just as the downstroke of the letter *p* is made; then the *e* is pronounced *ē* (as in the word *eat*) at the moment the downstroke of the letter *e* is made. The patient says nothing as he writes the final *a* of the word, because this *a* is a silent letter.

Note that the whispered *p* in *pea* is made exactly like the *p* in the word *pot*. For example, to say and write *pot* the patient whispers *p* on the downstroke of the letter *p*. He does not say the *p* as a letter of the alphabet (e.g., A & P stores). The *ŏ,* as in the word *hot,* is said on the downstroke of the *o;* and *t,* as in the word *foot,* is uttered on the downstroke of the letter *t*.

In case further questions arise as to how certain sounds are produced, make a careful study of one of the following phonetics texts: Wise, C. M., and Morgan, Lucia, *Progressive Phonetic Workbook* (William C. Brown Co., Dubuque, Iowa, 1948); West, Robert, and Kantner, Claude, *Kinesiologic Phonetics* (College Typing Co., Madison, Wisconsin, 1935).

Additional words which may be used to help the patient with writing and speaking are *hand, bell, rose, bed, key, bat, gun, cup, barn, bread, spoon, stove,* etc. See Drills 75–84 on pages 181–99. You will note that no vertical lines are included in Drills 81–84. If the patient has difficulty connecting the sound with the written word, he should practice the writing of these words with vertical lines before he does these drills. The therapist may prepare writing sheets for the words similar to those in Drills 72–80, on pages 175–91. Additional monosyllabic words which may be used are:

tie	bug	pie	cat	lamp	boat	crow
bed	car	bag	hill	dress	drape	back
hat	pen	rug	neck	rope	door	frog
man	toe	net	fork	belt	coat	plant
dog	cow	rat	wall	comb	horse	brush

At first it is better to write only monosyllabic words; then, later, two-syllable words may be used. Following are suggested words:

apron	eyebrow	lemon	razor
apple	eyelash	hammer	supper
arrow	finger	Mamma	water
candle	gravy	pencil	window

For additional suggestions see the text, Longerich and Bordeaux, *Aphasia Therapeutics,* pages 115–17.

In case the patient has marked difficulty integrating the speech and writing, it is better for him to say and write the sounds as separate units, e.g., *a r m,* but *think* of the sounds as a whole word. Later the sounds can be connected into the unified word, e.g., *arm*.

Usually, if a patient cannot pronounce a word aloud, he will have difficulty in writing it. It is,

© *Mary Coates Longerich 1955, 1958*

therefore, important that only words which the patient can articulate be selected for writing drill. Just as soon as the patient can say a word, e.g., *O, I,* the body parts, articles of clothing, etc. (see word list on page 11), work may begin in learning to write it. During the early days or weeks of aphasia therapy, it is usually better to write only one or two new words in each therapy session. Then, gradually, as the patient's abilities begin to develop, a greater number of words can be added. After the words *I, O,* and *no* have been learned, it is preferable to proceed next with concrete words. (See Drills 73–84, pages 177–99.) Abstract ideas are more difficult for the aphasic. After the patient has learned to say and write the names of approximately 50 concrete objects, begin on action words such as *rub, kick, walk, clap, wash,* etc. For additional suggestions, see the text, Longerich and Bordeaux, *Aphasia Therapeutics,* page 117.

With some patients it is helpful to practice writing words in sound groups:

h and	h at	p an
b and	b at	m an
l and	c at	c an
s and	m at	f an
	r at	

At this point some patients may wish to select new words for themselves to add to the sound groups. This drill will prove helpful to those patients who tend to confuse words that look alike, e.g., *was* and *saw; band* and *land;* etc. See Drills 93–97, pages 217–25.

Additional writing drills are as follows:

1. As soon as the patient has six or eight words in his speech-writing vocabulary, start giving him these same words to write from dictation. Pronounce the word aloud, and ask him to repeat it once or twice after you; then say and write the word as a unified process. It is often helpful to say the word aloud in unison with the patient as he writes it. See page 22. It is wise to have the patient do some writing from dictation at *each* practice session.

2. After the patient has developed some skill in writing single words from dictation, start using short phrases or sentences such as: *I eat bread; I go home; I see a bee.* Again have the patient repeat the sentence aloud after you have said it. Then, as soon as he has written a sentence and said it as a unified process, ask him to read it aloud to you. It is important that the patient do this with all his dictation, for in this way he is getting practice in reading aloud as well as in writing.

3. Sentences may be increased in length as the patient's writing ability improves.

4. When the patient is able to write more freely, dictate names, addresses, and telephone numbers and ask him to write them.

5. Give the patient some simple written or typed questions such as "Where do you live?" and ask him to write the answer. Gradually more difficult questions may be used.

6. When the patient is able to read aloud a simple paragraph, he may be asked to do so. Following the reading of it, he may be asked to write the answers to written or typed questions based on the content of the paragraph.

7. After the patient has 300 or 400 words in his speech-writing vocabulary, show him a picture such as may be found on the cover of the *Saturday Evening Post.* Give him the following directions, depending on his abilities:
    a. Write the names of the objects in the pictures.
    b. Read aloud the list of objects you have written.
    c. Tell several things that are happening in the picture.

© Mary Coates Longerich 1955, 1958

d. Write several ideas about the picture. Read aloud the sentences you have written.
e. Write a story about the picture. Read aloud what you have written.

It is understood that in all of the writing drills in this manual, the patient is to say and write every word as a unified process. Only by making this procedure consistent in *all* of the patient's writing can the desired results be obtained.

E. HELP WITH INDIVIDUAL SOUNDS
(For additional helps, see Longerich and Bordeaux, *Aphasia Therapeutics,* pages 139–48.)

Some patients may need very little help on the individual sounds, whereas others may require considerable drill. As the patient gains ability in imitating what he hears, there will be less need for work on individual sounds. Of course, some patients will need much more help than others. For this reason, the following lists of sounds are given as a guide in helping the patient:

m	Close the lips and hum. If the patient has difficulty making the sound, place your left index finger on the upper lip and your right index finger on the lower lip and guide his lips to the closed position. Say *m* as you close his lips.
b	Close lips and press them together. Say sound as you press the lips together.
p	Press lips together and whisper.
d	Push tip of tongue upward (behind upper front teeth) and say the sound. If the patient has difficulty lifting the tongue, use a tongue depressor to help him move it upward.
t	Push tip of tongue upward (behind upper front teeth) and whisper. If the patient has difficulty in lifting the tongue, use the tongue depressor as described for *d*.
n	Put tip of tongue upward as for *d* or *t* and "hum" with the lips open. If the patient has difficulty lifting the tongue, use the tongue depressor, as described for *d*.
l	Put tongue upward and sing *l* as in *la-la*. If the patient has difficulty lifting the tongue, use the tongue depressor, as described for *d*.
g	Press back of tongue against soft palate. Say the sound as you do this. In case the patient finds it difficult to make the sound, place the right thumb at the left upper edge of the patient's thyroid cartilage (i.e., Adam's apple) and the right index finger at the upper right edge of the thyroid cartilage. Press very lightly on the cartilage as you say *g*.
k	Press back of tongue against soft palate as for *g* and whisper. If the patient has difficulty saying *k*, proceed similarly as for *g*.
r	Tell the patient to say *ah;* then square his lips as he continues the sound. If he has difficulty in making the sound, suggest that he say *ah* then lift his tongue slowly. As soon as he can say *r*, have him omit the utterance of *ah*. Some patients find it easier to learn *r* by singing "Row, row, row, your boat." Tell the patient to square his lips as he says *row*.
z	Shut teeth and make the buzzing sound of a bee (*z-z-z-z*).

© *Mary Coates Longerich 1955, 1958*

s	Close teeth as for z sound and then whisper.
th (voiced as in *the*)	Place the tongue between the teeth and say sound.
th (voiceless as in *thick*)	Place the tongue between the teeth as for the voiced *th* and whisper.
sh	Round the lips. Close teeth and blow. It may help to have the patient think of the idea "Sh, be quiet" and place his fingers to his lips as if he is "shushing" someone.
y (as in *you*)	Press tongue downward and say the sound. Sometimes it helps to have the patient point to another person and emphatically say *you*.
w	Round the lips and say the sound. It may help the patient to tell him to make the sound of the wind, "woo!"
wh (as in *where*)	Round the lips as for *w* and whisper.
j (as in *judge*)	Shut the teeth. Press the tongue upward, round the lips slightly, and say the sound.
ch	Shut the teeth. Press tongue upward and round the lips slightly as for *j*, above, then whisper. It may help the patient to think of the sound of the engine "ch, ch, ch" in saying this sound.
ng (as in *sing*)	Press with back of the tongue against the soft palate. "Hum" with the lips open.
ah (as in *arm*, and the first part of the word *eye* [ah-ee])	Open mouth widely and then say the sound.
Long *o* (as in *ōld*)	Round lips and say the word.
oo (as in *mōōn*)	Round the lips as for *o;* then make the circle smaller.
e (as in *mē*)	Smile broadly and then say *ē*. If the patient has difficulty with this, it may help to tell him to lift the front part of his tongue.
Long *a* (as in *āche*)	Say *e* as in *me;* then open the mouth slightly.
Short *i* (as in *ĭt*)	Say long *e* as in *me;* then relax the lips slightly (in other words, smile a little less broadly).
Short *e* (as in *mĕt*)	Say short *ĭ;* then move lower jaw slightly downward.
Short *a* (as in *ăt*)	Say short *ĕ;* then move lower jaw slightly downward.
Short *o* (as in *nŏt*)	Say *ah;* then round the lips slightly.
oi, oy (as in *noise, boy*)	Say short *o;* then smile. Or, say short *o;* then add a short *ĭ*.
u (as in *hŭt*)	Move the lower jaw slightly downward.

The above suggestions are quite elementary. Usually it is easier for a patient to learn a sound within a meaningful word; e.g., long *i* can actually be learned when the patient is working on the word *eye*.

Consonants usually come more easily when they are followed by a vowel in a meaningful word: *bee*, *no*, *car*, *go*.

Again let it be emphasized that it is very important that the patient watch and *see* how sounds within words are produced. If he cannot imitate the sound, then he will need to be given specific suggestions for making the isolated sound.

F. SUGGESTED READINGS

Goldstein, Kurt: *Language and Language Disturbances.* Grune & Stratton, Inc., New York, 1948.

Granich, Louis: *Aphasia.* Grune & Stratton, Inc., New York, 1947.

Longerich, Mary C., and Bordeaux, Jean: *Aphasia Therapeutics.* The Macmillan Co., New York, 1954.

Nielsen, J. M.: *Agnosia, Apraxia, Aphasia.* Paul B. Hoeber, Inc., New York, 1946.

Weisenburg, T., and McBride, K.: *Aphasia.* The Commonwealth Fund, New York, 1935.

Wepman, Joseph M.: *Recovery from Aphasia.* The Ronald Press Co., New York, 1951.

Wise, C. M., and Morgan, Lucia: *Progressive Phonetic Workbook.* William C. Brown Co., Dubuque, Iowa, 1948.

© *Mary Coates Longerich 1955, 1958*

part three

DRILLS FOR THE PATIENT

A. DRILLS FOR RECEPTIVE APHASIA

DRILL 1

Directions (to the therapist): Give the patient a specific suggestion; then ask him to attempt it. Repeat the direction aloud at the moment the patient does the action. Frequently the patient will begin to say at least a word or two of the command in unison with the therapist. As soon as the patient can respond to one direction, give him two consecutive directions and ask him to try them. Again repeat the direction aloud as the patient performs it. If the patient is ambulatory, he may be given directions which require his moving about the room. Otherwise, he should be seated in front of a desk or table. Objects may be placed in front of him, and he may be asked to do certain things. Begin the drill by saying to the patient: "I shall tell you something I would like you to do; then I want you to do it." For example:

1. Point to your notebook.
2. Give me a pencil.
3. Show me the bookcase.
4. Point to the clock.
5. Give me the scratch pad.
6. Open the book.
7. Put your (left or right) hand on your head.
8. Close your eyes.
9. Open your eyes.
10. Point to the telephone.
11. Point to the floor.
12. Show me the window.
13. Open your notebook.
14. Close your notebook.
15. Snap your fingers.
16. Kick the desk.
17. Point to the ceiling.
18. Roll your pencil.
19. Point to your nose.
20. Point to the radiator.
21. Point to your mouth.
22. Place your hand over your eyes.
23. Point to your hair.
24. Scratch your neck.
25. Place the palm of your hand on the top of your head.

Twofold Directions:

26. Put your finger on your right ear and close your eyes.
27. Extend your arm and wave your hand.
28. Put your hand on your shoulder and make a fist.

(*continued on following page*)

DRILL 1 (*cont.*)

29. Lay your hand on your knee and spread your fingers.

If the patient is ambulatory, he may also be asked to do the following:

1. Open the door.
2. Close the door.
3. Turn off the light.
4. Turn on the light.
5. Put the pencil on the desk.
6. Stand up.
7. Open the window.
8. Close the window.
9. Knock on the door.

Twofold Directions:

10. Put your pencil on the chair and open the drawer of the desk.
11. Place the pencil on the desk and turn off the light.
12. Turn on the light and put the key in the ash tray.
13. Open your notebook and place it on the desk.

DRILL 2

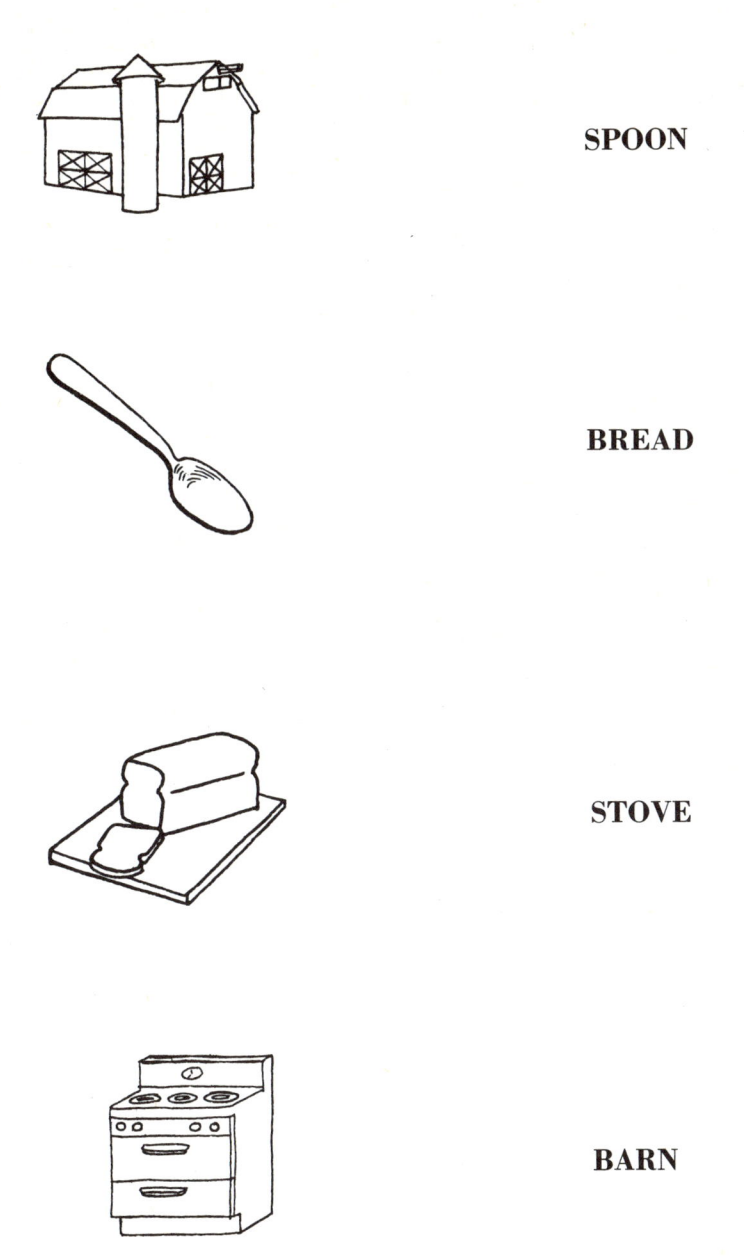

Directions (to be read to the patient by the aphasia therapist): Look at the objects at the left of the page. Then find the name of each object in the column at the right and draw a line to it.

SPOON

BREAD

STOVE

BARN

DRILL 3

Directions (to be read to the patient by the aphasia therapist): Look at the objects at the left of the page. Then find the name of each object in the column at the right and draw a line to it.

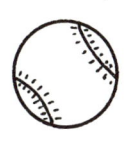

GUN

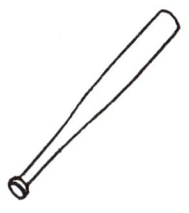

BALL

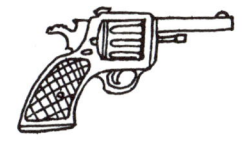

TENT

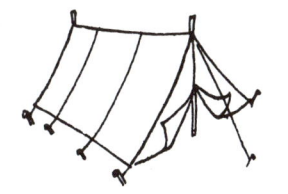

BAT

DRILL 4

Directions (to be read to the patient by the aphasia therapist): Read the words in the center column. Then find an object to which each word belongs. Draw a line from each word to its appropriate object.

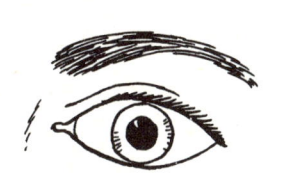

HAND

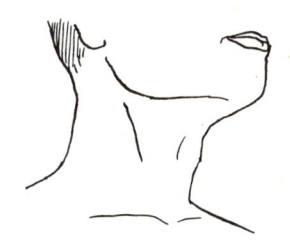

NOSE

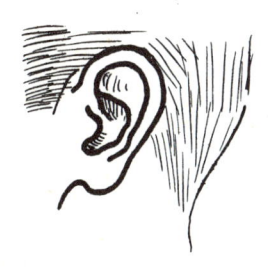

EYE

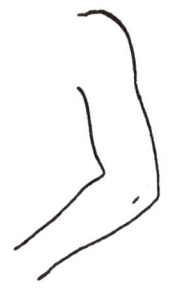

THROAT

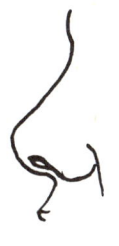

ARM

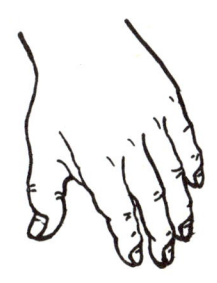

EAR

DRILL 5

Directions (to be read to the patient by the aphasia therapist): Look at each object. Then find the name of it among the words at the right of the picture. Draw a line from the object to the appropriate word.

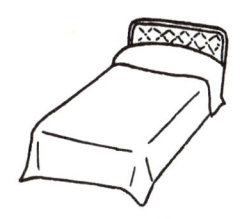

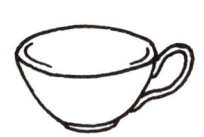

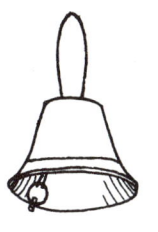

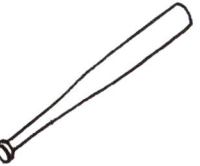

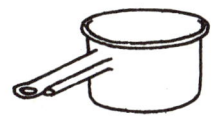

BID
BUD
BED
BAD

CAP
CAPE
CUP
COAT

BILL
BALL
BELL
BULL

BIT
BUT
BAT
BET

PANE
PAN
PEN
PIN

DRILL 6

Directions (to be read to the patient by the aphasia therapist): Read the words in each group at the left. Draw a circle around the word which is the name of the object at the right.

BRAID

BROAD

BREAD

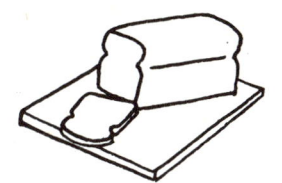

SPIN

SPOON

SPAN

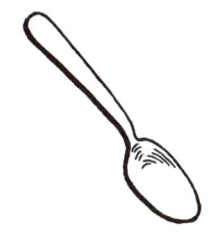

BRING

SING

RING

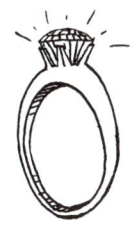

HOSE

ROSE

NOSE

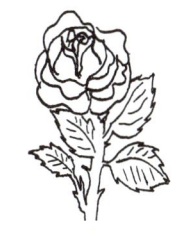

TENT

SENT

WENT

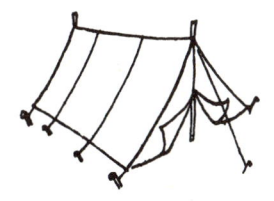

DRILL 7

Directions—review (to be read to the patient by the aphasia therapist): Look at each object on the page, name it, then find the suitable word for the object in the word list at the bottom of the page.

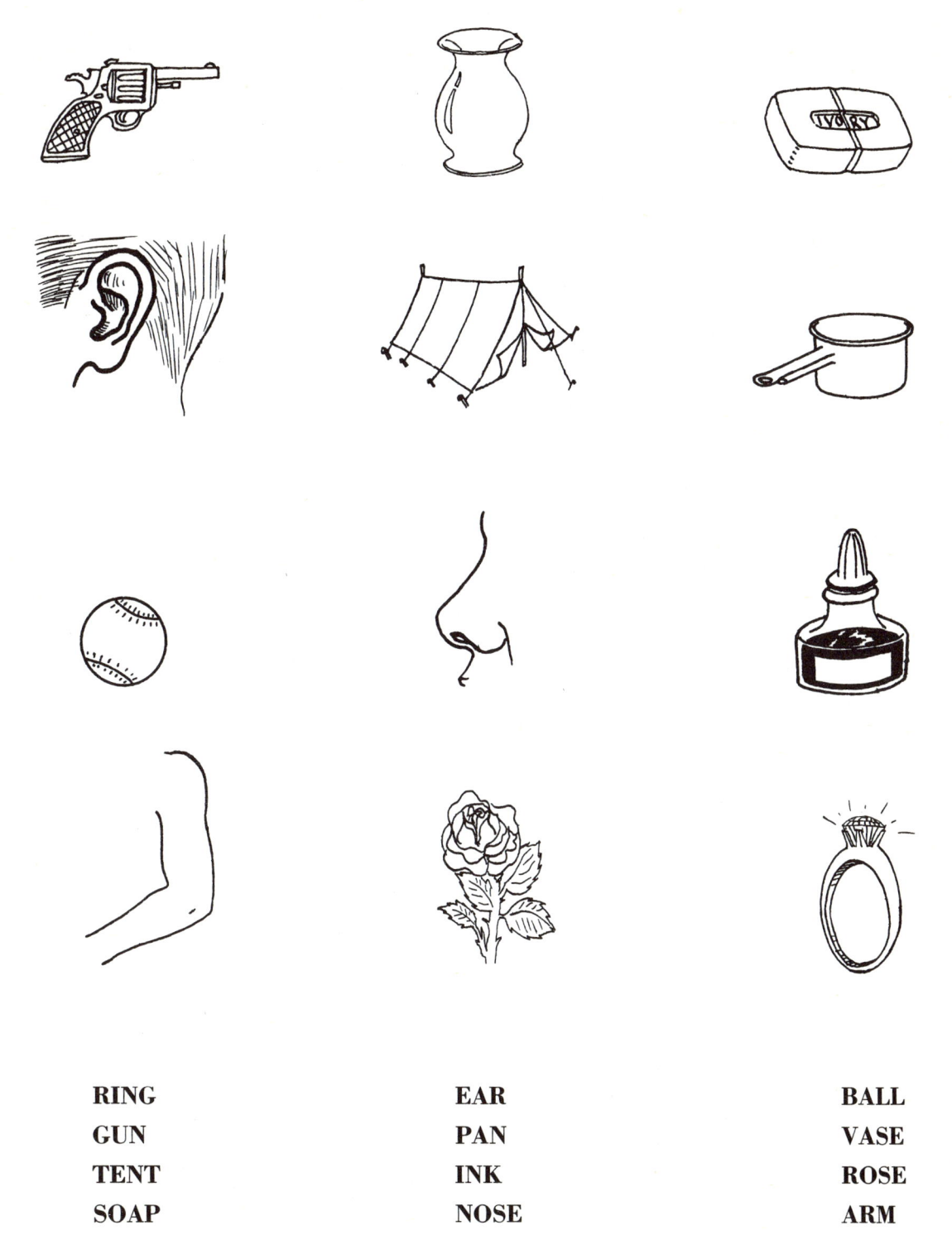

RING	EAR	BALL
GUN	PAN	VASE
TENT	INK	ROSE
SOAP	NOSE	ARM

43

© *Mary Coates Longerich 1955, 1958*

DRILL 8

Directions: Answer each question with *yes* or *no*.

1. Do you like steak? _____
2. Do you eat fish? _____
3. Do you use cream in your coffee? _____
4. Do you like to listen to the radio? _____
5. Do you like to see your friends? _____
6. Do you like rain? _____
7. Do you like to watch television? _____
8. Do you live in the United States? _____
9. Do you eat breakfast every morning? _____
10. Do you like candy? _____
11. Do you live in a city? _____
12. Are you a man? _____
13. Do you have a dog? _____
14. Do you like to swim? _____
15. Do you wear a wrist watch? _____

DRILL 9

Directions (to be read to the patient by the aphasia therapist): I shall read a group of questions. If a question is correct, answer *yes*. If it is wrong, say *no*.

1. Do trees grow?
2. Are newspapers good to eat?
3. Can a large steamer cross the ocean?
4. Can you smell a rose?
5. Can a cat bark?
6. Do oranges laugh?
7. Do houses walk?
8. Can a candle burn?
9. Do horses cry?
10. Can you eat eggs?
11. Do skunks smell good?
12. Can a dog sing a song?
13. Are apples good to eat?
14. Do birds fly?
15. Is sugar sweet?
16. Can bees fly?
17. Do babies jump rope?
18. Can you eat a chair?
19. Can fish swim?
20. Can a stove run?

DRILL 10

Directions: If a sentence is correct, write *yes* in the blank to the left of it. If it is false, write the word *no* in the space.

_____ 1. I am an American.

_____ 2. The sun sets in the east.

_____ 3. Texas is a large state.

_____ 4. Apples grow on vines.

_____ 5. The Pacific Ocean is east of the United States.

_____ 6. I am a farmer.

_____ 7. Canada is south of the United States.

_____ 8. The earth is flat.

_____ 9. Water is wet.

_____ 10. I like to eat.

DRILL 11

Directions: Read the following list of things you can see and do in the Los Angeles area. Write *yes* before the items you would enjoy; mark *no* before the ones you would not like.

_____ Visit Marineland.

_____ See the ships at the harbor.

_____ See the Pacific Ocean.

_____ Go to Disneyland.

_____ See the footprints at the Grauman's Chinese Theatre.

_____ See the movie stars' homes.

_____ See the Forest Lawn Art Objects.

_____ Go to a stage play.

_____ Go to a TV show.

_____ Go to the Farmers' Market.

_____ Eat at Knott's Berry Farm.

_____ Visit a movie studio.

_____ Go to church.

_____ Visit a university campus.

_____ See a football game at the Rose Bowl.

DRILL 12

Directions (to be read to the patient by the aphasia therapist): **Look at each of the objects on the page. Then draw a line to the name of the object in the center column.**

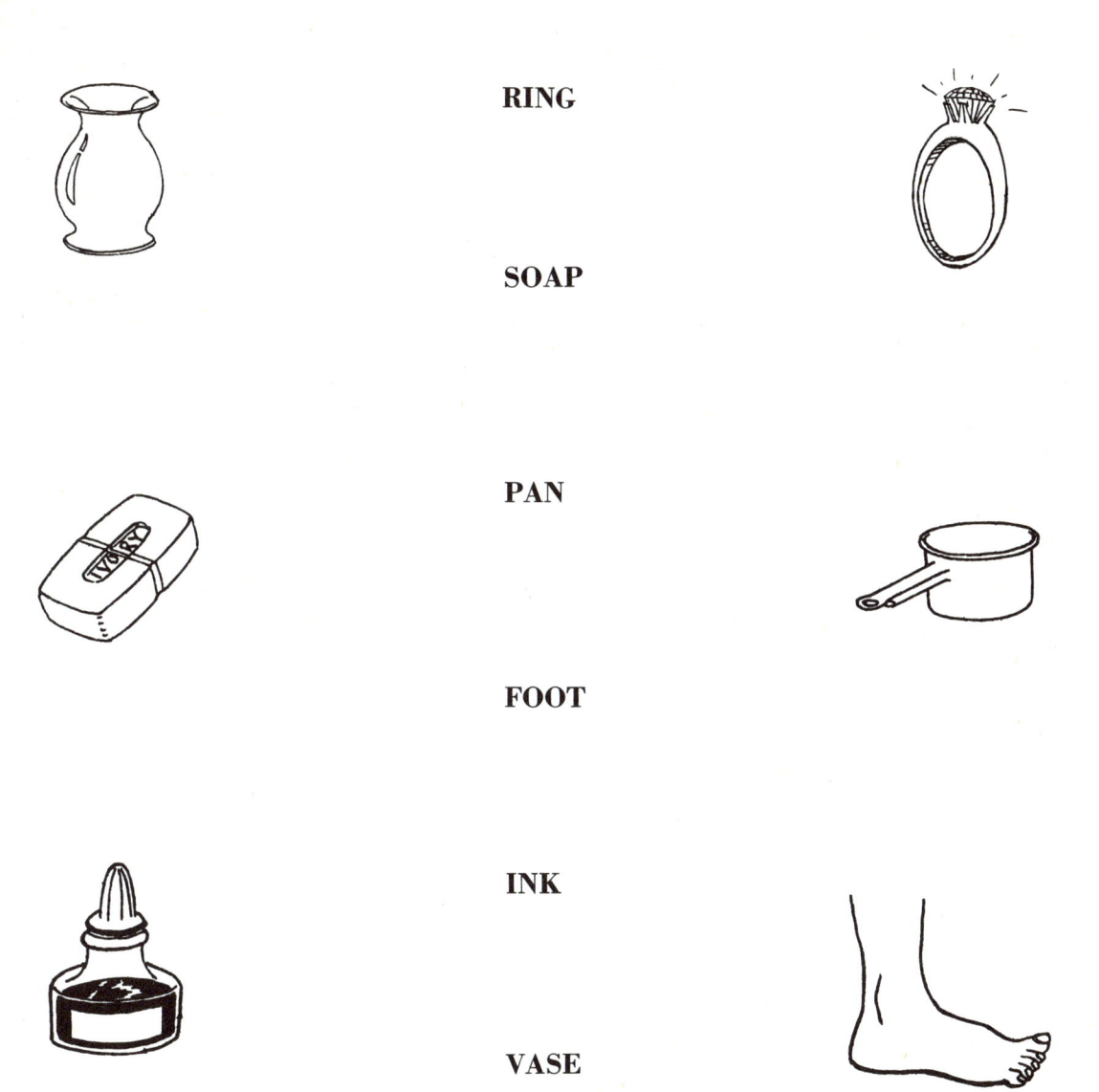

RING

SOAP

PAN

FOOT

INK

VASE

Directions (cont.): **I shall place a strip of paper over the words in the center column. Then I shall name each of the objects and you say the words with me if you can.**

DRILL 13

Directions (to be read to the patient by the aphasia therapist): Look at each object on the left side of the page. Then draw a line to the name of the object in the right-hand column.

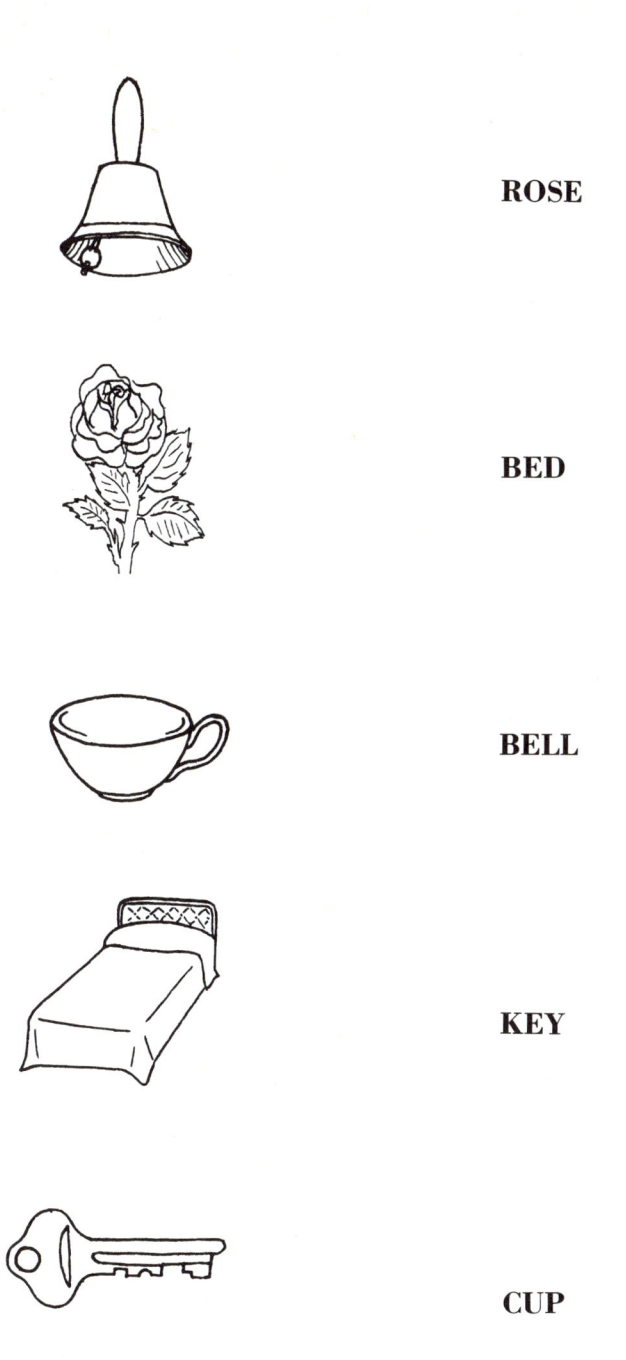

(bell)	**ROSE**
(rose)	**BED**
(cup)	**BELL**
(bed)	**KEY**
(key)	**CUP**

Directions (cont.): I shall place a strip of paper over the words in the right-hand column. Then I shall name each of the objects and you say the word with me if you can.

55

© *Mary Coates Longerich 1955, 1958*

DRILL 14

Directions **(to be read to the patient by the aphasia therapist): Read the words in the center column. Then draw a line to the appropriate object.**

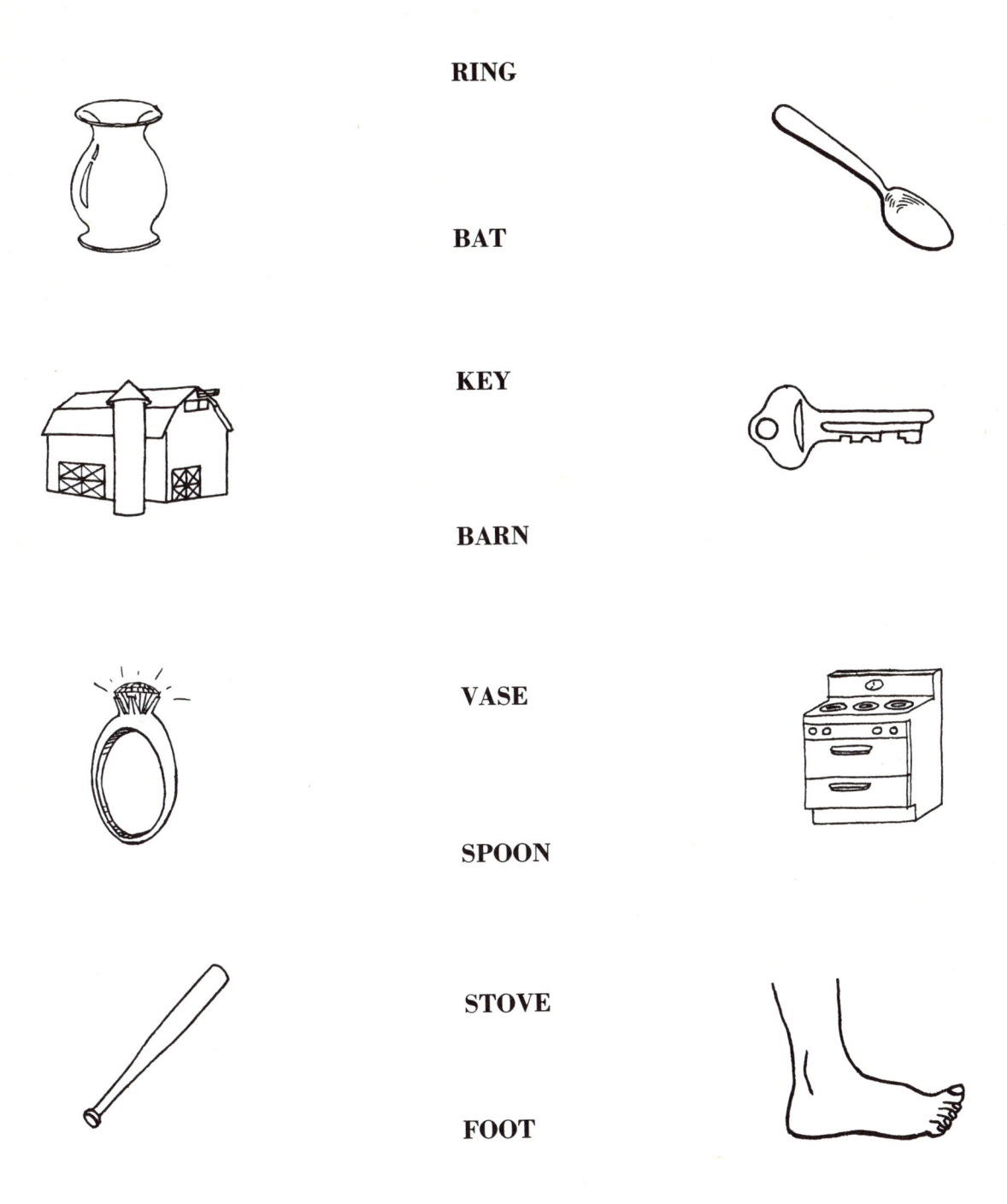

RING

BAT

KEY

BARN

VASE

SPOON

STOVE

FOOT

DRILL 15

Directions (to be read to the patient by the aphasia therapist): I shall read slowly some groups of numbers. After I read a group, you repeat the numbers after me.

4 — 2
8 — 3
2 — 7 — 4
3 — 1 — 9
4 — 2 — 5 — 7
3 — 1 — 6 — 2
8 — 4 — 7 — 3
9 — 2 — 1 — 5 — 3
8 — 1 — 4 — 7 — 6
1 — 4 — 8 — 6 — 9 — 2
1 — 2 — 3 — 9 — 5 — 7 — 4

DRILL 16

Directions:

Underline the words below which are the names of foods.

apples	steak
table	gravy
potatoes	lamp
radio	ice cream

Underline the words below which are the names of body parts.

ear	feet
chair	nose
toe	arm
hair	rose
beet	dog

Underline the articles used on a dinner table.

plate	knife
pillow	fork
spoon	cat
picture	napkin
child	wall

Underline the parts of a car.

engine	wheel
pear	spark plug
gun	windshield
hood	candle
coat	horn

DRILL 17

Directions: Mark a line through the incorrect answers.

1. Two things a nurse wears:
   uniform
   door
   gravy
   ice cream
   cap

2. Three things a man can do:
   gray
   sit
   run
   walk
   lamp

3. Four things an automobile has:
   engine
   desk
   steering wheel
   street
   horn
   sidewalk
   windshield
   river

4. Three things a man wears:
   belt
   shirt
   soap
   trousers
   meat

5. Two things a woman has:
   nose
   arms
   fins

6. Four things a maid uses for cleaning:
   soap
   television
   dust cloth
   broom
   vacuum
   radio
   telephone

7. Two things a girl can do:
   skip
   jump
   skill
   goat

8. Two things a kitchen has:
   stove
   hail
   refrigerator
   door
   mountain

(continued on following page)

DRILL 17 (cont.)

9. Three things a church has:
   organ
   bear
   minister
   stream
   steeple
   valley

10. Six things a dog can do:
    jump
    bark
    whine
    play
    fly
    sleep
    beg
    ski

11. Three things a bird has:
    wings
    dress
    beak
    feathers
    trees

12. Three things a baby does:
    fly
    sleep
    kick
    drive
    cry
    bark

13. Two things the ocean has:
    horse
    fish
    book
    water

14. Three things a house has:
    door
    tiger
    window
    river
    clouds
    wall

DRILL 18

Directions: Read the following word groups. Then select a suitable word in the box at the bottom of the page and write it at the left of each bracket. For example:

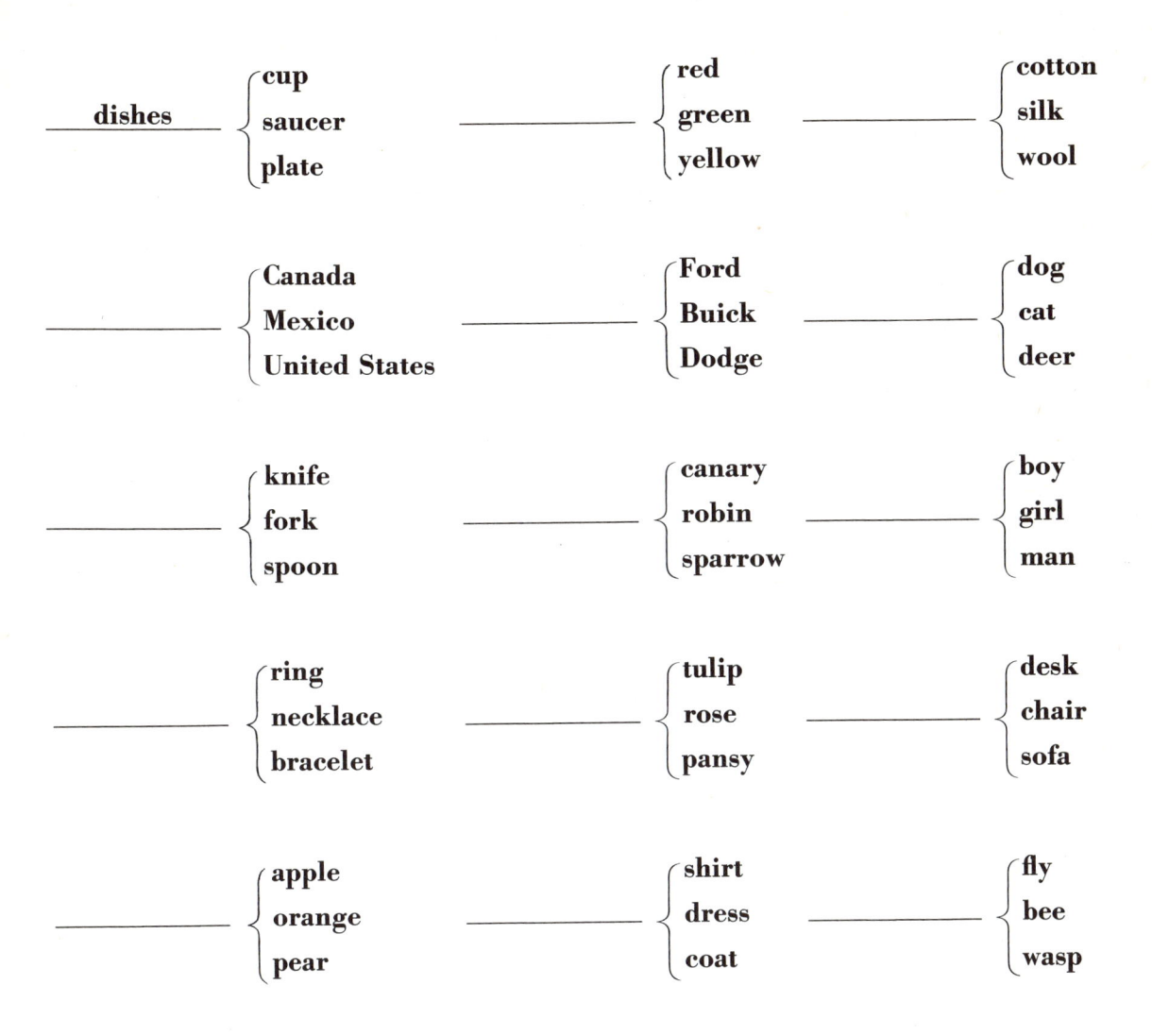

dishes { cup, saucer, plate }   _____ { red, green, yellow }   _____ { cotton, silk, wool }

_____ { Canada, Mexico, United States }   _____ { Ford, Buick, Dodge }   _____ { dog, cat, deer }

_____ { knife, fork, spoon }   _____ { canary, robin, sparrow }   _____ { boy, girl, man }

_____ { ring, necklace, bracelet }   _____ { tulip, rose, pansy }   _____ { desk, chair, sofa }

_____ { apple, orange, pear }   _____ { shirt, dress, coat }   _____ { fly, bee, wasp }

birds	insects	cars	silverware	furniture
people	jewelry	fruits	countries	colors
flowers	dishes	animals	clothing	materials

© *Mary Coates Longerich 1955, 1958*

DRILL 19

Directions (to be read to the patient by the aphasia therapist): Look at the words in each of the following word groups. I shall read aloud one of the words in each group and you point to the word I have read.

tree	coat	moon
see	boat	noon
bee	goat	spoon

win	pain	mill
tin	main	fill
pin	rain	will

bag	load	map
wag	toad	tap
rag	road	cap

DRILL 20

Directions: **Read the word at the first of the line. Draw a circle around the word every time it appears in the line.**

1. hat	but	hit	hot	bit	hat	bet	heat
2. now	not	never	new	now	nap	now	nod
3. bed	bad	did	deal	bed	bid	bed	deed
4. man	not	men	mine	mop	man	net	map
5. his	her	hip	his	hot	hop	his	hit
6. rat	rot	rate	rat	rut	run	ran	rat
7. pin	pan	pin	nap	pen	pin	pine	pane
8. saw	was	sew	sat	sir	saw	sit	sad

DRILL 21

Directions: Read the word at the top of each list. Then encircle the word every time it appears in the list.

<u>it</u>	<u>up</u>	<u>in</u>	<u>on</u>
is	on	is	up
by	up	on	no
no	by	by	us
at	up	in	of
it	no	up	on
on	is	no	by
up	us	an	is
an	of	in	on
are	up	at	an
it	is	in	on

DRILL 22

Directions: Look at the word in the left-hand column. Then find this word in the sentence to the right and underline it. For example:

dog	1. The <u>dog</u> ate the meat.
fish	2. Jack likes to fish.
friend	3. My friend is Bill Smith.
house	4. Tom and Jane have a new house.
cat	5. Mr. and Mrs. White have a black cat.
car	6. Jim has a new car.
lion	7. I saw a lion at the zoo.
window	8. The boy opened the window.
pie	9. Bill ate the pie.
horse	10. Bob likes to ride a horse.

DRILL 23

Directions: Read the list of words at the bottom of the page. Then find the word in each sentence and draw a circle around it.

Example: John is a (carpenter.)

1. Mrs. Jones is my grandmother.
2. I like to watch television.
3. Mr. Smith is an engineer.
4. I enjoy eating ice cream.
5. New York and Los Angeles are very large cities.
6. The Pacific Ocean is west of the United States.
7. Texas is a very large state.
8. Dogs make good pets.
9. Christmas is in December.
10. Ice skating is a winter sport.

carpenter	skating	television
grandmother	pets	enjoy
west	December	cities
state		engineer

DRILL 24

Directions (to be read to the patient by the aphasia therapist): I shall read aloud each of the phrases at the left side of the page. Then you read the words in the right-hand column and encircle the one that means almost the same as the phrase.

1. Part of a car.

    street
    wheels
    tree

2. The part of the body that contains the fingers.

    band
    hard
    hand

3. Part of a shirt.

    dollar
    collar
    hollow

4. Frozen water.

    ice
    ace
    rice

5. A garden plant with green leaves.

    garbage
    cabbage
    luggage

6. Something in which we sit.

    hair
    cheer
    chair

(continued on following page)

DRILL 24 *(cont.)*

		mining
7.	Part of a day.	mourning
		morning
		trio
8.	A large group of people.	audience
		guest
		wing
9.	Part of an airplane.	sing
		thing
		postman
10.	A type of car used for a train.	Pullman
		brakeman

DRILL 25

Directions: Read each word in the left-hand column. Then draw a line to its opposite in the right-hand column. For example:

on	hot	narrow	short
below	tight	lost	inside
cold	above	long	evening
happy	off	outside	wide
loose	sad	morning	found

many	hello	arrive	old
begin	go	often	thin
stop	dark	fat	slow
light	end	fast	leave
good-by	few	young	seldom

up	under	big	short
right	white	in	shiny
over	day	tall	light
night	left	heavy	little
black	down	dull	out

DRILL 26

Directions: **All but one of the words in each horizontal line rhyme. Find the word which does not rhyme and encircle it.**

1.	rod	nod	cod	pad	pod
2.	pole	male	sole	mole	role
3.	rap	hop	mop	stop	top
4.	beam	bean	dean	lean	mean
5.	maid	paid	raid	laid	file
6.	main	man	pain	gain	stain
7.	need	bleed	near	seed	weed
8.	hand	land	lend	band	sand
9.	pot	rot	pod	tot	hot
10.	think	rink	wink	sink	sunk

DRILL 27

Directions: All but two of the words in each of the following word groups rhyme. Encircle the two words which sound different.

feet	batch	rack
seat	latch	tuck
fat	witch	sack
beet	catch	pack
sheet	match	tack
set	ditch	lick
heat	hatch	lack

ten	bay	braid
pin	say	laid
men	day	paid
den	pan	toad
pan	ray	bowl
hen	bat	maid
pen	stay	raid

DRILL 28

Directions: Find three little words in each of the longer words. Write the little words on the lines at the right of the longer word.

1. lifesaver
2. sweetheart
3. landscape
4. tiresome
5. classmate
6. homeward
7. waterfall
8. handwriting
9. watchman
10. mankind
11. submarine
12. rainbow
13. photograph
14. bonfire

DRILL 29

Directions: **Encircle the little words which are contained in the longer words.**

                mailman

                headquarters

                eardrum

                carfare

                myself

                hatband

                mousetrap

                without

                dresser

                housewife

                garage

                doorstop

                endless

                favorable

                freeway

                bookshelf

                grandmother

                anteater

                friendship

                padlock

© *Mary Coates Longerich 1955, 1958*

DRILL 30

Directions: Read each of the following words. Then find the little words in each of the bigger words. Write three little words to the right of the big word.

1. butterflies _____ _____ _____
2. gentleman _____ _____ _____
3. tomorrow _____ _____ _____
4. unbutton _____ _____ _____
5. fireplace _____ _____ _____
6. carefully _____ _____ _____
7. dripping _____ _____ _____
8. together _____ _____ _____
9. something _____ _____ _____
10. visitor _____ _____ _____
11. candlelight _____ _____ _____
12. wherever _____ _____ _____
13. appointment _____ _____ _____
14. typewriter _____ _____ _____
15. wondering _____ _____ _____
16. arrangement _____ _____ _____

DRILL 31

Directions: **Underline two little words in each of the following big words.**

1. salesman
2. seashore
3. watchman
4. chairman
5. railway
6. pancake
7. teaspoon
8. forehead
9. cowboy
10. homesick
11. innkeeper
12. fisherman
13. sunlight
14. rosebud
15. armchair
16. bedroom
17. nightgown
18. pathway
19. lighthouse
20. sidewalk
21. horseback
22. bathrobe
23. airplane
24. rainfall
25. landlord
26. platform
27. waterfall
28. limestone
29. whenever
30. cobweb

DRILL 32

Directions: Read the underlined word at the top of each list. Then try to find this "little" word in each of the words in the list. Some of the words will contain the little words, and some will not.

<u>hen</u>	<u>at</u>	<u>ill</u>	<u>is</u>
then	hat	fill	his
when	shatter	roller	listen
Wednesday	station	still	this
Henry	stop	million	history
apprehension	into	till	fist
helmet	attitude	well	hasten
them	operator	mill	list

<u>it</u>	<u>or</u>	<u>oil</u>
military	for	core
itself	transport	coil
fit	draw	sore
still	card	soiled
hitting	airport	cord
butter	resort	tinfoil
situation	pillow	boil

DRILL 33

Directions: Read each of the following words. Then find the little words in each of the bigger words. Write three little words below each big word.

1. milkman
   _____
   _____
   _____

2. steamboat
   _____
   _____
   _____

3. livingroom
   _____
   _____
   _____

4. toothbrush
   _____
   _____
   _____

5. cannot
   _____
   _____
   _____

6. snowplow
   _____
   _____
   _____

7. firecracker
   _____
   _____
   _____

8. attendance
   _____
   _____
   _____

9. snapshot
   _____
   _____
   _____

10. grandfather
    _____
    _____
    _____

11. baseball
    _____
    _____
    _____

12. sunshine
    _____
    _____
    _____

13. important
    _____
    _____
    _____

14. policeman
    _____
    _____
    _____

15. bumblebee
    _____
    _____
    _____

16. discover
    _____
    _____
    _____

DRILL 34

Directions: Read aloud the two groups of words below. Observe that the "oy" in the list at the left side of the page is pronounced exactly like "oi" in the words at the right side of the page.

oy	oi
boy	oil
toy	boil
joy	toil
Roy	coil
	spoil

Now read the sentences and underline the words containing the "oy" or "oi" sound.

1. Roy is a tall boy.
2. Jim has a new oil well.
3. The workmen toil for many hours.
4. The water will boil soon.
5. I will not let the food spoil.
6. The baby was happy to have a new toy.
7. I wound the wire in a coil.
8. Roy put oil in his car.
9. Cream may spoil in hot weather.
10. The cat liked his toy mouse.

DRILL 35

Directions: Read aloud the words in the list below. Then read the sentences and underline the words which contain the "ow" or "ou" sound. Note that "ow" and "ou" are pronounced exactly alike.

GROUP A

cow	owl	gown	brown	power
now	fowl	town	frown	tower

GROUP B

out	loud	round	south	our
pout	cloud	found	mouth	hour

1. I went to town today.
2. The ball team will go south this winter.
3. Ed Brown found an owl in the barn.
4. Our house is one mile south of town.
5. I see a cloud in the sky.
6. The farmer lost his cow.
7. I hear a loud bell.
8. Bill found a baseball.
9. He fell on a brown rock.
10. I hear the loud motor of the car.
11. Tom has a new brown ball.
12. I will go to the tower of the building.

DRILL 36

Directions: Read aloud the words in the two lists. Note that the "aw" and the "au" in each of the lists are pronounced exactly alike.

aw	au
law	Paul
raw	haul
saw	fault
caw	
jaw	
straw	

Complete each of the following sentences by using one of the words from the above list.

1. The man will _____ the hogs to town.
2. I _____ my doctor at the movie today.
3. The thief broke the _____ .
4. I do not like _____ carrots.
5. It is not my _____ that I am late.
6. The boxer received a broken _____ .
7. The crow began to _____ .
8. He drank his soda through a _____ .
9. A policeman will keep _____ and order.
10. _____ is a man's name.

DRILL 37

Directions: **Read aloud the following words. If you have difficulty, you may review the previous exercises which contained these words.**

fault	found	joy
town	saw	south
spoil	power	oil
Paul	coil	owl
joy	fowl	straw
caw	loud	cow
frown	mouth	boil
law	cloud	tower
haul	jaw	gown
out	now	round
brown	pout	toil
raw	hour	our
Roy	toy	boy

DRILL 38

Directions: Read a word in the left-hand column. Then draw a line to its related word in the right-hand column. For example:

read	**television**
drink	**coat**
eat	**newspaper**
smoke	**milk**
ring	**lunch**
button	**bell**
watch	**cigarette**

DRILL 39

Directions: Read each of the words in the left-hand column. Then draw a line to the word in the right-hand column which represents a part of it. For example:

1. foot   drawer
2. knife   word
3. fork   oven
4. sentence   toe
5. face   leaf
6. car   finger
7. stove   beak
8. hand   yolk
9. tree   chin
10. desk   blade
11. egg   prong
12. bird   wheel

© Mary Coates Longerich 1955, 1958

DRILL 40

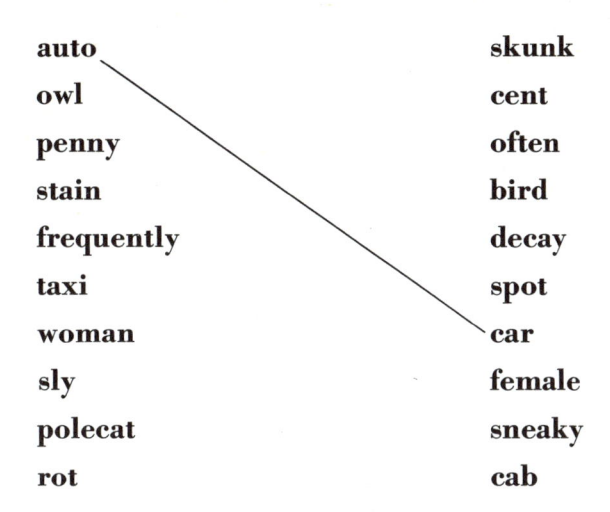

Directions (to be read to the patient by the aphasia therapist): Read each of the words in the left-hand column. Then draw a line to the word with a similar meaning in the right-hand column. For example:

auto	skunk
owl	cent
penny	often
stain	bird
frequently	decay
taxi	spot
woman	car
sly	female
polecat	sneaky
rot	cab

DRILL 41

Directions (to be read to the patient by the aphasia therapist): Read the words below. Then place each word at the left of the phrase which means approximately the same thing (see example 1).

lion	hostess	county
tire	party	coin
tree	nest	Canada
	car	

_____lion_____ 1. A wild animal.

_____ 2. A piece of money.

_____ 3. A rubber covering of an automobile wheel.

_____ 4. A country north of the United States.

_____ 5. Something which has leaves.

_____ 6. One who entertains in her home.

_____ 7. A social gathering.

_____ 8. A bird's home.

_____ 9. An automobile.

_____ 10. A part of a state.

DRILL 42

Directions (to be read to the patient by the aphasia therapist): Read each of the following phrases. Then select a word from the bottom of the page which means approximately the same as the phrase. Write the word in the space at the left of the phrase.

_____ 1. Before noon.

_____ 2. Not false.

_____ 3. Come face to face.

_____ 4. A man who marches.

_____ 5. Money paid for the use of a house.

_____ 6. A large body of water.

_____ 7. Once more.

_____ 8. What is worn on the foot.

_____ 9. A slow-moving animal.

_____ 10. Rub out.

_____ 11. A nickname for William.

_____ 12. Wet, soggy earth.

soldier	again	meet	turtle
true	morning	mud	Bill
shoe	rent	sea	erase

DRILL 43

Directions (to be read to the patient by the aphasia therapist): Read each of the phrases in the left-hand column. Then find a word that corresponds to it in meaning in the right-hand column. Write the word at the left of the phrase.

_____	a. Served as President of the U.S.	bed
_____	b. Sound of a crow.	Jane
_____	c. A girl's name.	arrive
_____	d. Upper House of Congress.	nose
_____	e. To reach where you started to go.	caw
_____	f. A day of the week.	pen
_____	g. Something on which you sleep.	Sunday
_____	h. Something on which you write.	county
_____	i. A month of the year.	April
_____	j. A big monkey.	paper
_____	k. An organ of smell.	Theodore Roosevelt
_____	l. A body of still water.	ape
_____	m. Something with which you write.	pond
_____	n. Part of a state.	Senate

© Mary Coates Longerich 1955, 1958

DRILL 44

Directions: Read the words at the left of the page. Then find a phrase in the list at the right of the page which resembles each of the words in meaning. Place the number of the phrase in the space at the left of each word.

_____ chair	1.	A woman who cares for a house.
_____ refrigerator	2.	A person who flies an airplane.
_____ mechanic	3.	A woman who sews.
_____ maid	4.	Someone who cuts hair.
_____ Mexican	5.	Something we sit on.
_____ secretary	6.	A person who takes care of teeth.
_____ food	7.	A person who types.
_____ chef	8.	One who repairs a car.
_____ pilot	9.	A man who cooks.
_____ seamstress	10.	Someone from Mexico.
_____ barber	11.	Something we eat.
_____ dentist	12.	A man who performs on the stage or in the movies.
_____ author	13.	Something in which we store food to keep it fresh.
_____ pajamas	14.	Something we wear to bed.
_____ actor	15.	A person who writes books, plays, or articles.

DRILL 45

Directions: Write the correct word in the space. Then read the sentence aloud. For example:

	to
1. John has ___two___ cars.	two
	too
	read
2. The American flag is _____ , white, and blue.	red
	write
3. Bill throws a ball with his _____ hand.	right
	noise
4. The dog has a big _____ .	nose
	hire
5. Jane has very pretty _____ .	hair
	tar
6. The cat caught the _____ .	rat
	urn
7. We must work to _____ a living.	earn
	dear
8. The hunter shot a _____ .	deer

(continued on following page)

DRILL 45 (*cont.*)

9. The child _____ his horn.

blew

blue

10. The diamond in her ring is _____ .

reel

real

DRILL 46

Directions: Read the two words at the left of each sentence. Then select the correct word to write in the blank. For example:

gain, game   1. Bill will go to the football ____game____ .

window, winds   2. Jack _____ the clock before he goes to bed.

horse, house   3. Jane and Peg will go to the _____ races today.

saw, sew   4. Sally likes to cook and _____ .

ran, rain   5. Bob likes to walk in the _____ .

frog, four   6. I saw a _____ near the river.

beat, bear   7. I saw a deer and a _____ at the zoo.

door, dong   8. I will open the _____ for you.

dish, fish   9. I like to eat _____ .

window, wind   10. Bill will open the _____ .

DRILL 47

Directions: Read aloud the three words at the left of each sentence. Then select the correct one and insert it in the blank.

need

weed   1. The man will _____ chains on his tires.

seed

mole

male   2. The boy had a big _____ on his face.

role

land

hand   3. The farmer hurt his _____ on his plow.

sand

hot

pot   4. The cook dropped the _____ plate on the floor.

pod

man

main   5. Mr. Jones is a very fine _____ .

pain

sink

sunk   6. The maid will clean the _____ .

wink

(continued on following page)

DRILL 47 (cont.)

laid

paid   7. John must _____ his tax report.

file

wink

think   8. Do you _____ it will rain today?

rink

need

near   9. Bill lives _____ the lake.

weed

pad

pod   10. Jim and Tom caught some _____ fish.

cod

DRILL 48

Directions: Read the three underlined words below. Then select which word should be used in each of the sentences.

<u>wash</u>　　　　　　　　<u>washed</u>　　　　　　　　<u>washing</u>

1. I am _____ my hair.
2. I _____ my clothes yesterday.
3. I _____ my hands before I eat.
4. Have you _____ your car?
5. Are you going to _____ the dishes?
6. Bill _____ his dog in the tub.
7. The doctor _____ his hands well.
8. The man will _____ the windshield of my car.
9. The maid _____ the windows last week.
10. The man will _____ the tile floor.

DRILL 49

Directions: Read each of the sentences below. Then find a word at the bottom of the page to complete each sentence.

1. The rabbit ate a _____ carrot.
2. The men will _____ the corn to market.
3. Bill _____ the lawyer for his services.
4. This is _____ raincoat.
5. I shall _____ the steaks in the oven.
6. The car rolled _____ the hill.
7. I _____ when I am in the bright sun.
8. The fisherman must always take _____ when he goes fishing.
9. The food will _____ in the warm car.
10. Tom _____ his tie clasp in the grass.
11. I eat when I am _____ .
12. John received his _____ from high school.

down   hungry
raw   your
diploma   found
frown   paid
bait   broil
spoil   haul

DRILL 50

Directions: Draw a line through the word which is incorrect.

1. Bill has a new top (cat, coat).
2. I have to (feed, fed) the bird.
3. I think it will (rain, ran) today.
4. I broke the (steam, stem) of the rose.
5. The (mean, men) will build the bridge.
6. I (paid, pad) for my dinner.
7. This is a (steep, step) hill.
8. I wrote the note on the (paid, pad).
9. I wash my hands with (sap, soap).
10. The boy will run to the (goal, gal) post.
11. I shave with my (zoo, razor).
12. I eat with my (frock, fork).

DRILL 51

Directions: **Read the sentences below and then choose the correct words.**

1. Maud asked me to _____ the paint in the can.

    shirt

    stir

2. The woman got some _____ on her shoes.

    skirt

    dirt

3. The doctor is a _____ person.

    kind

    find

4. The carpenter has _____ his work today.

    none

    done

5. Jim is a new teacher at the _____ .

    stool

    school

6. The soldiers are standing in a straight _____ .

    dine

    line

7. We will keep _____ at Lake Arrowhead.

    cool

    fool

8. The boys showed _____ of the lions at the zoo.

    clear

    fear

(*continued on following page*)

DRILL 51 (cont.)

9. The enemy made a _____ on our camp.

raid

paid

10. I gave my wife a gold _____ for her dress.

pin

bin

DRILL 52

Directions: Read the two words at the left of each sentence. Then select the suitable word to write in the blank space.

hollow, follow	1. The dog likes to _____ his master.
cottage, cotton	2. The old man lived in a _____ on the hill.
poppy, popcorn	3. I like to eat _____.
gobble, bottle	4. I will buy a _____ of olives.
chopping, hopping	5. The farmer is _____ down the tree.
offer, office	6. The doctor is sitting in his _____.
proper, polish	7. Jane will _____ the silver.
collar, coral	8. The dog lost his _____.
offend, officer	9. I saw the police _____.
dollar, donkey	10. I had to pay a _____ for parking in the lot.

DRILL 53

Directions: Read the following list of words. Then find a word in the list that will make each sentence correct.

gone	do
one	does
on	say
no	said
saw	
was	

1. Bill and his girl have _____ to the movies.
2. I have _____ use for snowshoes in Southern California.
3. Tom _____ leaving for the wedding at seven o'clock.
4. I _____ not want cream in my coffee.
5. _____ it rain very often in Oregon?
6. The maid _____ she needed more soap for the laundry.
7. I _____ a jet plane.
8. Bob has only _____ car for his big family.
9. Did you _____ you would be here at ten o'clock?
10. Sue put _____ her sunglasses when she walked along the beach.

DRILL 54

Directions: The two words at the end of each sentence look very much alike. Encircle the word which should be used to complete the meaning of the sentence.

1. The man shot ducks in the (stream, scream).
2. The students ate a hearty (mean, meal).
3. The farmer had a large flock of (steep, sheep).
4. The dentist filled the man's (tree, teeth).
5. As the fireman climbed out of the window, he tore his (boots, boats).
6. The car salesman gave his customer a fair (dean, deal).
7. The framework of a car is made of (seal, steel).
8. John is captain of his basketball (tray, team).
9. We shall have our lunch at (noon, room).
10. The airline stewardess served dinner to the people on the (pane, plane).

DRILL 55

Directions: **Read the sentences below and underline the correct word. For example:**

1. The man will (eat, <u>read</u>) the paper.
2. Bill will come home at (room, noon).
3. The hunter carried his (gun, pun).
4. I like to watch the (moon, soon) in the sky.
5. The sailors like to go to (seat, sea).
6. The child had (fear, pear) of the dog.
7. I must (wind, mind) the clock tonight.
8. The sun shines in the (sty, sky).
9. The child fell on the (scare, stair).
10. This is a very (tool, cool) day.
11. Jane will (cake, take) me to the store.
12. I do not like the (beat, heat) in the summer.
13. Tom lives (bear, near) Seal Beach.
14. I will sit in the (hair, chair).
15. I shall buy a (fair, pair) of socks.

DRILL 56

Directions: Underline the correct word.

1. Bob (work, **worked**) forty hours last week.
2. The bird in the cage is (sing, **singing**).
3. Sally (**baked**, bake) a pie for her boy friend.
4. Bill lost his two (**tickets**, ticket) to the boxing match.
5. The boy (whistle, **whistles**) for his dog.
6. The mother (look, **looked**) for her little girl.
7. The show (last, **lasts**) for two hours.
8. It (mist, **mists**) sometimes on a cloudy day.
9. Jim (call, **called**) for me at nine o'clock.
10. Bill does not have (**another**, other) ticket left in his taxi book.

DRILL 57

Directions: Read the following sentences and insert the appropriate word.

1. The dog _____ the little boy's leg. (bit, bat)
2. Jack sat in the back _____ of the theater. (seat, sit)
3. George received a _____ and pencil for his birthday. (pen, pan)
4. Bill _____ the ball with his left hand. (lit, hit)
5. The woman will try not to get too _____ . (fat, bat)
6. Bob likes to eat _____ for lunch. (neat, meat)
7. Jane forgot to _____ the clerk for her groceries. (pit, pay)
8. The two _____ were playing tennis. (man, men)
9. The farmer pitched the _____ into the loft. (hay, heat)
10. The cat _____ down the street. (can, ran)
11. The football players felt their team would be hard to _____ . (beat, bit)
12. John _____ the oven of the stove. (hit, lit)
13. I _____ swim under water. (cat, can)
14. Helen is a _____ housekeeper. (meat, neat)
15. Everyone should vote on election _____ . (day, hay)

DRILL 58

Directions: Read aloud the two words at the right-hand side of the page. Then select the one which you should use to make the sentence read correctly.

1. Jack ate his _____ .

    dinner

    dining

2. Bill _____ to his dog.

    whistle

    whistles

3. The telephone is _____ .

    ring

    ringing

4. John caught a big _____ .

    fishing

    fish

5. Tom will help me _____ the furniture.

    move

    moves

6. The gardener is _____ the lawn.

    waters

    watering

7. A doctor must have many years of _____ .

    schools

    schooling

8. I think Bob will win the school _____ .

    elected

    election

(*continued on following page*)

DRILL 58 (cont.)

9. Sue says she _____ bake a cake.

will

mill

10. Babies do a lot of _____ .

crying

cries

11. Mr. Jones _____ his fence.

painted

painting

12. We _____ television until ten o'clock.

watches

watched

13. The water in the teakettle is _____ .

boils

boiling

14. Dick likes to _____ golf.

play

playing

15. The Browns are planning to _____ to Europe this summer.

travels

travel

DRILL 59

Directions: Read the words at the right of each sentence. Then select the word which will complete the sentence and write it in the blank space.

1. Harry _____ a mile this morning. walked, walking

2. Mother is _____ the milk for our cat. warm, warming

3. Mr. Jones is _____ some Ford stock today. buys, buying

4. Bill _____ baseball at Westlake Park yesterday. played, playing

5. The train will be _____ Los Angeles at two o'clock. leaves, leaving

6. Sally has _____ flowers to her mother every week. bringing, brought

7. The dog always _____ at a loud noise. barks, barking

8. Tom is _____ his car in front of the house. stopping, stops

9. Bill _____ today for his fishing trip. starts, starting

10. Mother _____ us every summer. visits, visiting

DRILL 60

Directions: Underline the word which will correctly complete the sentence.

1. I must put a (damp, stamp) on a letter before I mail it.
2. Mrs. Jones sent her son to the store to get a loaf of (bread, bead).
3. A man wears shoes and (locks, socks).
4. I wear a rain (cat, coat) when it rains.
5. A man shaves with a (radar, razor).
6. I always take my fishing (rod, cod) when I go fishing.
7. The dog fell into the (sake, lake).
8. The truck driver sometimes sleeps during the (bay, day) and does his driving at night.
9. The carpenter must always have his (toads, tools).
10. Bill goes to work on the (bus, puss).
11. I try to keep (tool, cool) on hot summer days.
12. A teacher goes to (stool, school) each morning.
13. The sun shines in the (sky, sty).
14. The little girls like to (made, wade) in the pool.
15. The streets are (met, wet) after a rainstorm.

DRILL 61

Directions: Draw a circle around the word which will correctly complete the sentence.

1. We look at the clock to see the (time, mine) of day.
2. A dog wags his (sail, tail) when he is happy.
3. We like a (drink, brink) of water if we are thirsty.
4. The musicians gave a (comfort, concert) tonight.
5. There is not a (cloud, crowd) in the sky on a clear day.
6. The little boy began to (try, cry) when he dropped his ice cream cone.
7. The filing cabinet is made of (petal, metal).
8. We must pull down the (shades, shaves) in order to darken the room.
9. The gardener watered the (lawn, fawn).
10. The teacher showed her students a (nap, map) of the United States.
11. The mother will bake her little girl a birthday (rake, cake).
12. The kitten has soft (fur, far).
13. The fastest way to travel is by (plane, flame).
14. When it snows, the ground is (might, white).

DRILL 62

Directions: Underline the word which makes the sentence read correctly.

1. (Us, We) eat dinner at six o'clock.
2. This is (you, your) hat.
3. Please give (me, my) a pencil.
4. They will come to (our, they) home for lunch.
5. This is (you, your) chair.
6. He lost (he, his) billfold.
7. Where do (you, your) live?
8. (They, It) is warm today.
9. (They, Our) are going to Florida.
10. (Our, Us) car is in the driveway.

DRILL 63

Directions: **Encircle the suitable word in each of the sentences.**

1. He lost the button off (his, her) vest.
2. He drove (her, his) wife's car to town.
3. She lost (his, her) earring.
4. He took (his, her) wife to the play.
5. She gave (her, his) husband a birthday gift.
6. He got (his, her) haircut and shave at the barbershop.
7. He removed (her, his) hat when he entered the doctor's office.
8. She asked (her, his) husband for some candy.
9. She borrowed some paper from (his, her) husband's secretary.
10. He helped (her, his) wife into the car.

DRILL 64

Directions: Read the words in the list below. Then select an appropriate word from the list to complete each sentence.

his	my
your	her
their	our

1. The football players will get _____ new letters today.

2. Jane lost _____ purse at the store.

3. We shall get _____ new car today.

4. Did you lose _____ earrings?

5. Bill will get _____ award today.

6. Would you like me to lend you _____ pen?

7. The dog lost _____ collar.

8. Are you going to take _____ camera to the picnic?

9. We shall get _____ fishing licenses before we leave.

10. The twins Bill and Tom went to meet _____ father at the airport.

11. Sue will have _____ purse repaired at the leather shop.

12. This is _____ reel and fishing rod; that one is Tom's.

DRILL 65

Directions: Read aloud the first part of each sentence. Then underline an appropriate phrase at the right to complete the meaning.

1. If your room is cold, you should

    eat candy.
    turn on the heat.
    watch television.

2. If you are hungry, you should go

    to the movie.
    to the restaurant.
    to the gas station.

3. If you are sleepy, you should

    sing.
    go to bed.
    eat a steak.

4. If you are tired, you should

    laugh.
    rest.
    work faster.

5. If you are thirsty, you should

    get a drink of water.
    wash your teeth.
    blow a horn.

6. If you are ill, you should see a

    veterinarian.
    doctor.
    tailor.

7. If you want to buy cigarettes, you should go to the

    church.
    drugstore.
    hospital.

DRILL 66

Directions: Write a sentence, using each of the following groups of words.

1. States   in   I   United   the   live
   _____

2. fish   like   men   to   the
   _____

3. today   bake   Jane   cake   a   will
   _____

4. shot   boy   rabbit   the   a
   _____

5. porch   man   sat   a   on   the
   _____

6. hair   brown   the   has   man
   _____

7. knife   little   his   lost   the   boy
   _____

8. clock   I   a   see   big
   _____

9. bed   a   sleep   I   in
   _____

10. lunch   noon   eat   I   at
    _____

DRILL 67

Directions: Read each of the following word groups. Then formulate them into a sentence.

1. is going   Jack   this summer   to the beach

2. is repairing   Bill Jones   in his car   the motor

3. to college   John   medicine   will go   to study

4. a concert   to hear   we are going   tonight

5. don't like   some dogs   a bath   to have

6. clothes   her own   to make   Janet   likes

7. ice cream and cake   at the party   ate   the boys and girls

8. enjoy taking   Bob and Sally   of the children   movies

9. to swim   his little brother   taught   Frank

10. hoped   be elected   he would   the candidate

DRILL 68

Directions: Read each of the following lists of words and formulate them into a sentence.

1. knock   I   door   on   the   will
   _____

2. today   laid   men   the   carpet   the
   _____

3. zoo   Jack   went   and   to   Bill   the
   _____

4. house   week   painted   Jim   his   last
   _____

5. poet   Longfellow   a   great   was
   _____

6. car   I   for   gasoline   need   the
   _____

7. freezer   Sue   electric   new   a   has
   _____

8. six   eat   o'clock   dinner   I   evening   at   every
   _____

9. park   dog   I   to   my   the   took
   _____

10. pansies   sidewalk   near   planted   the   I
    _____

part three

DRILLS FOR THE PATIENT (*cont.*)

B. DRILLS FOR EXPRESSIVE APHASIA

DRILL 69

Directions (to be read to the patient by the aphasia therapist): I shall name the objects below, and you try to say them with me if you can.

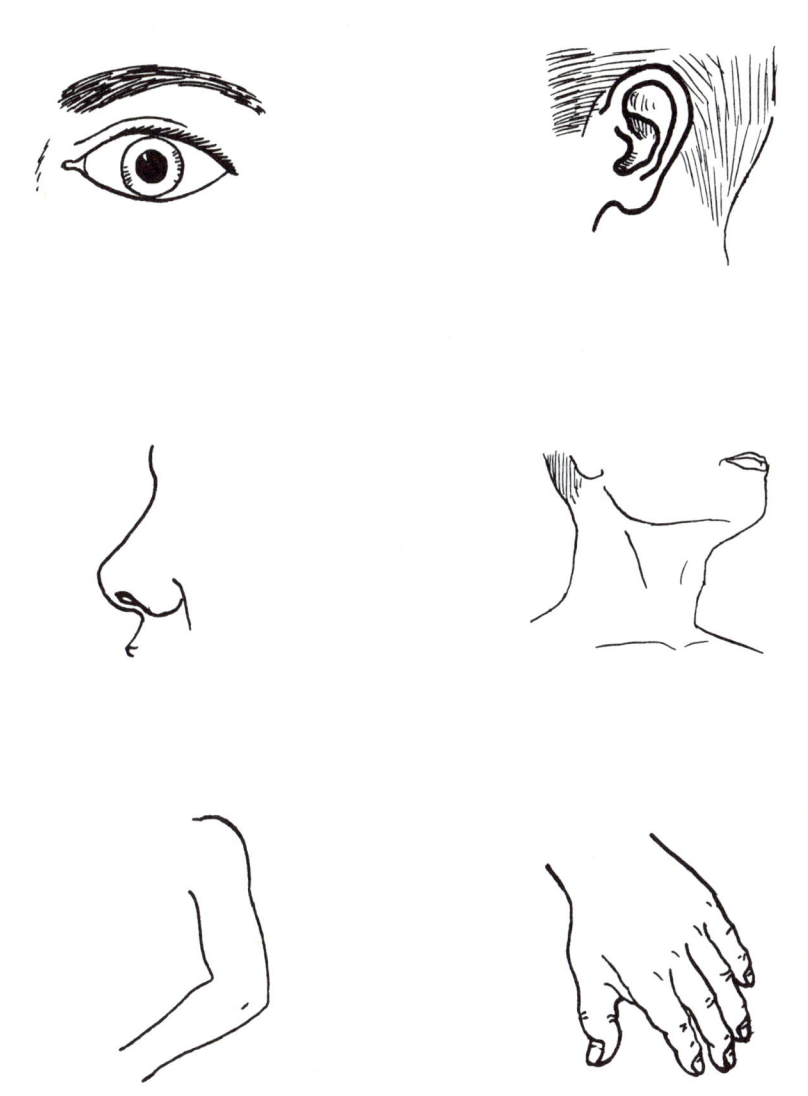

DRILL 70

Writing 𝒪

DRILL 71

Writing ℓ

ℓ ℓ ℓ

DRILL 72

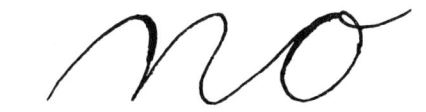

Writing no

DRILL 73

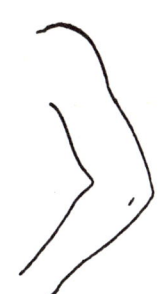

Writing

arm arm

DRILL 74

Writing

* *ear   ear   ear*

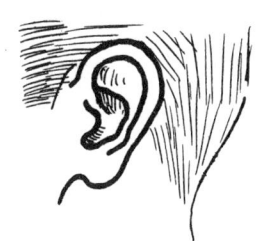

---

* A line is marked through the *a* to indicate it is a silent letter.

DRILL 75

Writing

nose   nose

* A line is marked through the *e* to indicate it is a silent letter.

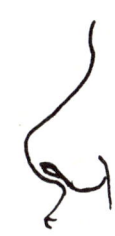

DRILL 76

Writing

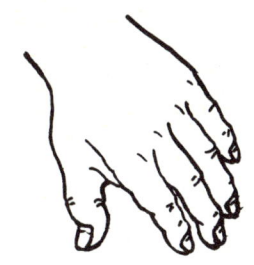

hand   hand   hand

DRILL 77

Writing

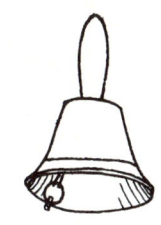

bell   *bell*   *bell*

DRILL 78

Writing

*rose   rose   rose

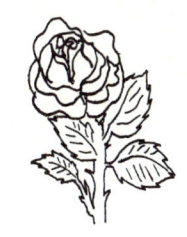

* A line is drawn through the *e* to indicate it is a silent letter.

DRILL 79

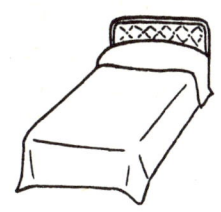

Writing

bed *bed* *bed*

DRILL 80

Writing

key   *key*   *key*

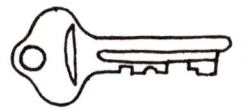

* A line is drawn through the *y* to indicate it is a silent letter.

DRILL 81

Directions (to be read to the patient by the aphasia therapist): Read the words at the bottom of the page. Then find an object below to which each word belongs. Write the suitable word three times at the right of the picture. Make certain you write and say the word as a unified process.

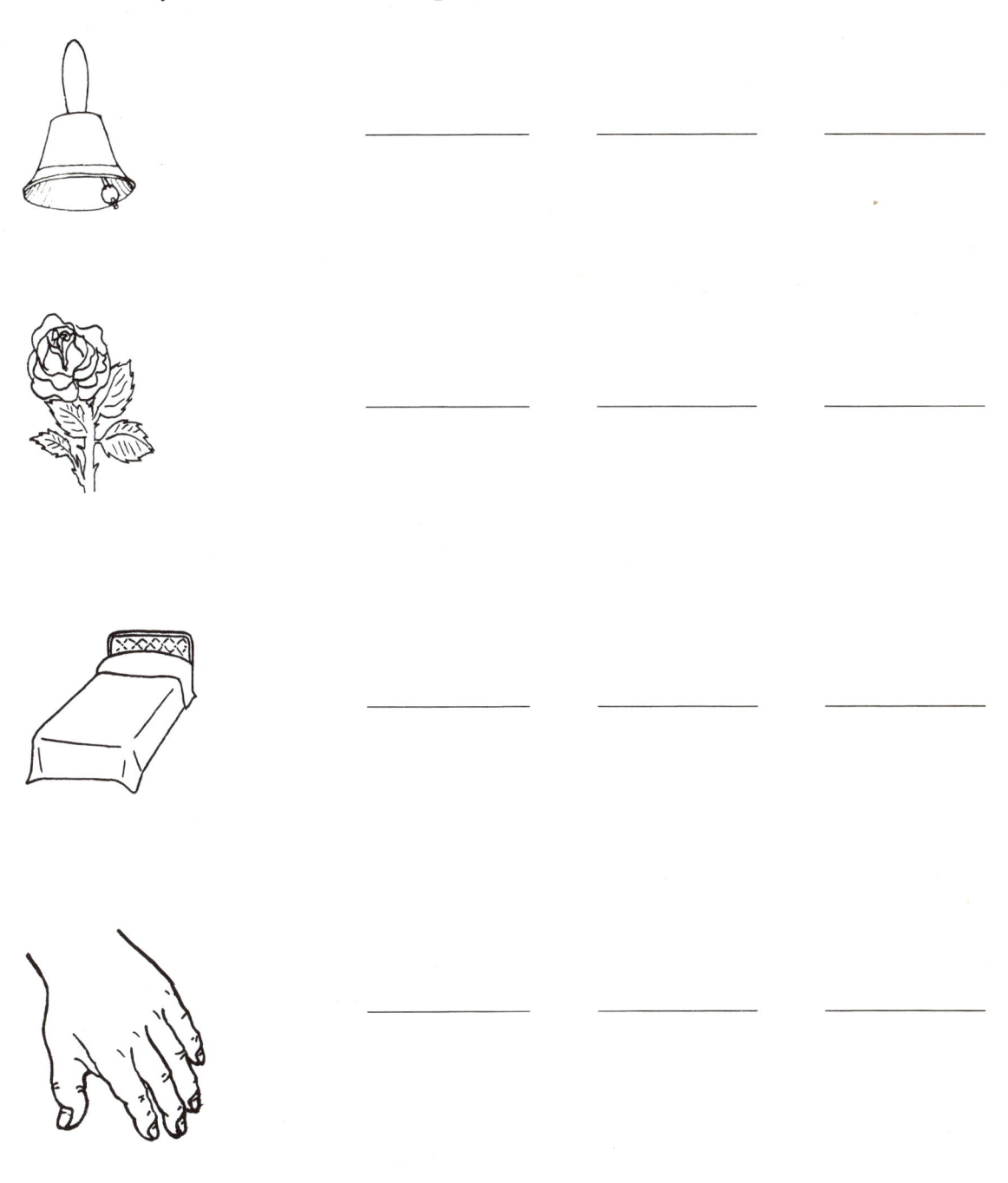

    ROSE   **HAND**   **BED**   **BELL**

DRILL 82

Directions (to be read to the patient by the aphasia therapist): **Read the words in the list below. Then look at each object and find the name of the object in the word list. Write the name three times on the lines to the right of the picture.**

KEY   HAND   BED   FOOT   ARM

_____

_____

_____

_____

_____

195

© *Mary Coates Longerich 1955, 1958*

DRILL 83

Directions (to be read to the patient by the aphasia therapist): I shall name each of the objects on this page and you say the word with me if you can.

CUP	**GUN**	**KEY**
TENT	**BAT**	**BALL**

Directions (*cont.*): Look at each of the objects. Then find its name in the list above. Write the word four times below the picture.

DRILL 84

Directions (to be read to the patient by the aphasia therapist): I shall name each object on the page, and you say the word with me if you can. Later you will write the name of the object four times at the right of the picture.

DRILL 85

Directions: Read the sentences in unison with your therapist. Then read them aloud by yourself.

1. Hello.
2. How are you?
3. I'm fine.
4. Please sit down.
5. Thank you.
6. You're welcome.
7. Give me a drink of water, please.
8. It's a nice day.
9. Please pass me the salt.
10. I'm hungry.
11. Let's eat dinner.
12. Good-by.
13. How do you do?
14. Excuse me.
15. Good morning.
16. Good evening.
17. What is it?
18. All right.
19. Where are you going?
20. Good night.

DRILL 86

Directions (to be read to the patient by the aphasia therapist): I shall perform several actions. As soon as I do something, you tell me what I am doing. For example:

ACTION	RESPONSE
1. Knocking on the table.	1. Knocking on the table, knock on the table, hit the table, etc.
2. Opening the door.	
3. Closing the door.	
4. Tapping with a pencil.	
5. Whistling.	
6. Erasing.	
7. Humming.	
8. Snapping finger.	
9. Rolling pencil.	
10. Opening the book.	
11. Tapping foot.	
12. Opening the drawer.	
13. Closing the drawer.	
14. Writing.	

DRILL 87

Directions (to be read to the patient by the aphasia therapist): I shall read the first part of a sentence to you. Then you supply the missing word.

1. I like ice cream and _____.
2. The sun shines during the _____.
3. The moon shines at _____.
4. Wisconsin is on the 10-yard _____.
5. I drink coffee with sugar and _____.
6. A fish _____.
7. Grass is _____.
8. Three cheers for the red, white, and _____.
9. I drink _____.
10. I wash my hands with _____.
11. Row, row, row your _____.
12. Birds _____.
13. I eat with a _____.
14. I drink water out of a _____.
15. We ride in a _____.
16. Cows give _____.
17. A cat catches _____.
18. A window is made of _____.
19. A chair is made of _____.
20. I write with a _____.

DRILL 88

Directions (to be read to the patient by the aphasia therapist): I shall read a list of words. After I read each word, you tell me its opposite. For example, when I say <u>good</u>, you will reply <u>bad</u>.

up	—	down
long	—	short
left	—	right
stop	—	go
in	—	out
good	—	bad
over	—	under
hard	—	soft
true	—	false
black	—	white
lost	—	found
above	—	below
night	—	day
beginning	—	end
rough	—	smooth
inside	—	outside
fat	—	thin
big	—	little
happy	—	sad
light	—	dark
morning	—	evening
shallow	—	deep
far	—	near
loose	—	tight
narrow	—	wide
sweet	—	sour

DRILL 89

Directions: Read the first word of each line. Then write two additional words which rhyme with the first one. For example:

1. sat   <u>bat</u>   <u>cat</u>
2. cut
3. big
4. pan
5. bug
6. hog
7. top
8. dot
9. pin
10. did
11. ham
12. pet
13. tap
14. bad
15. cub

DRILL 90

Directions (to be read to the patient by the aphasia therapist): I shall give you a word such as pie. Then I want you to tell me a word that will rhyme with it. For example, tie.

1. Name a food that rhymes with lake.
2. Name a bird that rhymes with row.
3. Name an animal that rhymes with hat.
4. Name a flower that rhymes with lazy.
5. Name an article of furniture that rhymes with hair.
6. Name a number that rhymes with do.
7. Name a bird that rhymes with howl.
8. Name a color that rhymes with bed.
9. Name a beverage that rhymes with silk.
10. Name a color that rhymes with stew.
11. Name a tree that rhymes with coke.
12. Name an article of clothing that rhymes with mouse.
13. Name a kitchen utensil that rhymes with man.
14. Name a coin that rhymes with time.
15. Name a season that rhymes with call.

DRILL 91

Directions: **Read each of the following words. Then write each one below the word with which it rhymes.**

rag	rank	crab	sent
hip	tap	down	flake
dish	felt	mouse	fled
sand	tin	camp	bank

1. tag
   _____

2. melt
   _____

3. house
   _____

4. bent
   _____

5. sank
   _____

6. bed
   _____

7. lip
   _____

8. gown
   _____

9. rake
   _____

10. fish
    _____

11. grab
    _____

12. lap
    _____

13. hand
    _____

14. grin
    _____

15. lamp
    _____

16. tank
    _____

DRILL 92

Directions: Write at least three rhyming words below each of the following words.

1. ride

2. bay

3. bone

4. hat

5. ran

6. race

7. date

8. bit

9. pail

10. had

11. nut

12. hid

13. bake

14. tame

15. pine

DRILL 93

Directions: Read these sound families.

hen	man	bat	bit	seat	bay
den	ran	cat	hit	meat	day
ten	can	sat	lit	beat	may
men	fan	fat	sit	heat	hay
pen	pan	mat	pit	neat	pay

The words in the above sound families appear in the list below. Try to read the entire list. In case you have difficulty, look for the word you are trying to say in its sound family at the top of the page. This most likely will help you to read the difficult words.

pen	pan
hay	day
seat	neat
lit	man
can	beat
mat	pit
bit	cat
pay	bay
ran	den
hen	hit
hat	fan
sit	heat
meat	may
ten	sat
fat	men

DRILL 94

A. *Directions:* In the following list encircle the words which begin with the humming sound *m*.

wind	wake
way	mill
make	will
wet	want
more	made
watch	wall
mitt	merry
wade	mud
wit	walnut
met	wood

B. *Directions:* Read the words in the following list, e.g., <u>will-mill</u>. Keep in mind that you form your lips in a small circle for *w* and that you close your lips for the humming sound *m*.

will	—	mill
we	—	me
wade	—	made
wet	—	met
wit	—	mitt
way	—	may
wake	—	make
wore	—	more

DRILL 95

Directions: Read the following word groups; for example, big-dig. Observe that the *b* and *d* sounds look very much alike. The *b* is made by putting your lips together, whereas the *d* is said by placing your tongue tip on the ridge just behind your upper teeth.

bay	—	day
big	—	dig
bill	—	dill
bare	—	dare
bean	—	dean
bell	—	dell
ban	—	Dan
bet	—	debt
bait	—	date
bad	—	Dad
bid	—	did
buck	—	duck

DRILL 96

Directions: Read the following word groups. Note that the first word in each pair looks very similar to the second. Be very careful to read the words forward; for example, saw not was.

saw	—	was
pot	—	top
nap	—	pan
mad	—	dam
dog	—	God
loop	—	pool
pit	—	tip
not	—	ton
rat	—	tar
lap	—	pal
pat	—	tap

DRILL 97

Directions: **Read the following word groups; for example: <u>mill</u>-<u>will</u>-<u>fill</u>. Remember that you close your lips for** *m*; **make a small round lip opening for** *w*; **and "bite" your lower lip for** *f*.

mill	—	will	—	fill
may	—	way	—	Fay
mow	—	woe	—	foe
mail	—	wail	—	fail
more	—	wore	—	four
mind	—	wind	—	find
mitt	—	wit	—	fit

DRILL 98

Directions: Read the phrase at the left side of the page. Then read its corresponding contraction at the right side of the page.

I am	—	I'm
I do not	—	I don't
I will	—	I'll
I cannot	—	I can't
I have	—	I've
I would	—	I'd
Is is not?	—	Isn't it?
I will not	—	I won't
He has not	—	He hasn't

Read each of the contractions in the left column. Then write its complete meaning in the space at the right.

1. He won't _____
2. They haven't _____
3. We won't _____
4. She doesn't _____
5. She hasn't _____
6. They can't _____
7. We aren't _____
8. It isn't _____
9. They weren't _____
10. You didn't _____

DRILL 99

Directions: Answer each question with *yes* or *no*. Place your answer in the space following the questions.

1. Are your lips on your face? _____
2. Can you open the window? _____
3. Has a house a tail? _____
4. Is your leg on your face? _____
5. Has a cat five feet? _____
6. Can you sit at a desk? _____
7. Can a dog bark? _____
8. Can you close your eyes? _____
9. Does a house have ears? _____
10. Is five more than eight? _____
11. Can you carry a fishing rod? _____
12. Can you bake a cake? _____
13. Can a car laugh? _____
14. Can a horse eat? _____
15. Can you tell me your first name? _____
16. Are your toes on your feet? _____

DRILL 100

Directions: **Read the questions and underline the correct answer.**

1. Can a cat bark?	YES	NO
2. Is New York east of California?	YES	NO
3. Do cows sing?	YES	NO
4. Do monkeys have feathers?	YES	NO
5. Can you feel the wind?	YES	NO
6. Do you eat with a fork?	YES	NO
7. Is it ten o'clock?	YES	NO
8. Is a rat a mouse's mother?	YES	NO
9. Does a hen have three legs?	YES	NO
10. Are ripe apples green?	YES	NO
11. Is ice cream black?	YES	NO
12. Do ducks swim?	YES	NO
13. Can you light a match?	YES	NO
14. Do you put salt on your watermelon?	YES	NO
15. Does the sun rise in the east?	YES	NO

DRILL 101

Directions: Read the anecdote. Then answer the questions.

On Sundays, the college boys who work with Bill in the campus cafeteria do not have to do so many chores as on week days. They have to prepare dinner at noon, but they do not have to wash the tables and floors. When the noon dinner is completed, the boys scrape the dishes and stack them. Then, their work is over for the day. Bill and his friend Tom usually go swimming. Some of the boys go into Denver to see the sights, while others just stay around the campus and loaf for the remainder of the day.

1. Where does Bill work?

    _____ in Denver; _____ in the campus cafeteria

2. Which meal do the college boys have to prepare?

    _____ breakfast; _____ dinner

3. Do the boys have to scrub the floors on Sunday?

    _____ yes; _____ no

4. What is Bill and Tom's usual pastime on Sunday?

    _____ going to Denver; _____ swimming

5. What is a suitable title for this story?

    _____ Cafeteria Duties on Sunday; _____ Eating on Sunday

DRILL 102

Directions: Read the anecdote. Then answer the questions.

One afternoon Noah Webster was entertaining the maid in the kitchen when suddenly Mrs. Webster opened the door. Horrified at seeing her husband making love to the servant, she exclaimed, "Well! I'm surprised!" "Oh, no, my dear," Webster replied, "You're amazed; I'm surprised."

1. Where was the maid?

2. Who was entertaining her?

3. Who suddenly walked into the kitchen?

4. How did Mr. Webster feel?

DRILL 103

Directions: Read the anecdote. Then answer the questions.

One noon the singer Ethel Merman went to an open-air restaurant in Central Park, New York, for luncheon. When she had ordered a fruit salad and started to eat, her dog Hansel began begging for food. Knowing that Hansel would have little interest in her salad, she was puzzled to know what to do. In a moment, a man at her right got up from his table. Seeing that a whole lamb chop had been left on his plate, she felt it shouldn't be wasted. So immediately she reached over to get it for Hansel. Just as the dog was taking his last licks on the bone, to Miss Merman's dismay the man returned to his table and found no lamb chop—not even the bone! The man had gone to answer the telephone.

1. Where was Ethel Merman having luncheon?

    _____ Chicago; _____ New York

2. What did she order?

    _____ lamb; _____ fruit salad

3. Who begged her for food?

    _____ Hansel; _____ a man

4. What did the man leave on his plate?

    _____ a drum stick; _____ a lamb chop

5. Why did the man leave the table?

    _____ to pay his check; _____ to answer the telephone

DRILL 104

Directions: Read the anecdote. Then answer the questions.

One afternoon the comedian Jack Benny made a $5 bet with a man on a baseball game. When Mr. Benny lost, the man asked him to autograph the bill, then proceeded to explain to Mr. Benny that his grandson wanted to frame the bill and keep it as a souvenir. "You mean the money is not going to be spent?" asked Mr. Benny. "Yes, that's correct." "Well," said Mr. Benny, "then I'll just write you a check."

1. On what kind of a game did Jack Benny make a bet?

    _____ football game; _____ baseball game

2. How much of a bet did he make?

    _____ $5; _____ $10

3. Who won the bet?

    _____ Jack Benny; _____ the man

4. What did Jack Benny decide to do?

    _____ go to New York; _____ write a check

DRILL 105

Directions: **Explain how to:**

1. Light a cigarette.
2. Sew on a button.
3. Clean your glasses.
4. Squeeze orange juice.
5. Set a table for company.
6. Fix a tire.
7. Bake a cake.
8. Tune in a TV program.
9. Set the alarm of an alarm clock.
10. Fix coffee.
11. Milk a cow.
12. Feed a dog.

DRILL 106

Directions (to be read to the patient by the aphasia therapist): I shall read some questions to you and I want you to answer them.

1. What direction would you have to face so that your right arm would be toward the west? (south)
2. What direction would you have to face so that your left arm would be toward the north? (east)
3. What direction would you have to face so that your left arm would be toward the east? (south)
4. Imagine that you are facing east; then you turn right. What direction would you then be going? (south)
5. Imagine that you are facing north; then you turn to your right; then you turn to your left. In what direction would you then be going? (north)
6. Imagine that you are facing west; then you turn right; then you turn left; then you turn left again. In what direction would you be going? (south)
7. Imagine that you are facing north; then you turn left; then you turn right; then you turn right again; then you turn left. In what direction are you going? (north)
8. Imagine you are facing north. You turn right; you turn left; you turn left again. What direction are you facing? (west)
9. Imagine you are facing west. You turn right; you turn right again; you turn left; you turn left again. What direction are you facing? (west)
10. Imagine you are facing east. You turn left; you turn right; you turn left; you turn left again; you turn right. What direction are you facing? (north)

DRILL 107

Directions (to be read to the patient by the aphasia therapist): Tell what is absurd about each of these statements.

1. An old lady said, "I'm no longer able to take my walk around the block every day. I can just go half way around and back again. That's all!"
2. Jane received a party invitation from her girl friend which contained this final statement: "If you don't receive this note, let me know and I'll send you another invitation."
3. In Greece there are two relics of the apostle Paul: one is his skull when he was nine years old and the other is his skull when he was a grown man.
4. The comedian said: "I'm really not conceited; I don't believe I'm half as funny as I really am."
5. There is a tree in North America so tall that it requires two adults and a child to see the top of it.
6. This morning, I met a good-looking, middle-aged man. He was walking down the street with his hands in his pockets and was twirling a shiny new cane.
7. A circus placed an ad in a newspaper which read: "Wanted: a dwarf and a giant." An old man of average height applied for the job and stated that he could play both parts. "You see," he said, "I'm the smallest giant in the world and the biggest dwarf."
8. The brakeman fell from the train and broke his neck, but received no further injury.
9. Betty and Janet lived several blocks from each other. It was getting dark and they were afraid to walk home alone. "I have a good idea," said Betty. "First I'll walk home with you and then you can walk home with me."

DRILL 108

Directions (to be read to the patient by the aphasia therapist): I shall read a statement. Then you tell me what is absurd about it.

1. An old farmer saw an advertisement in the paper: "Purchase a Fowler stove and save half of your coal." The farmer decided to buy two stoves in order to save all of it.
2. A private, drilling at boot camp, said that every soldier was out of step except himself.
3. A professor made the following announcement to his students: "On Friday of this week we'll have a test, attendance at which is voluntary; so if any student is absent, beware! You may get an 'F'."
4. My wife read in the newspaper that a burglar fired two shots at Mr. Jones. The first shot killed Mr. Jones, but the second one didn't.
5. When there is a train wreck, frequently the last car receives the most damage. Now I think it would be a good idea for the last car to be taken off before the train ever starts.
6. An old man said to the cobbler: "Stupid! I told you to make one of these boots bigger than the other. Instead you made one of them smaller than the other."
7. Bill is thin and Jim is thin, but Tom is thinner than both Bill and Jim put together.
8. An Englishman went to the post office and asked if they had a letter for him. The postmaster said, "What's your name, sir?" The Englishman replied, "Oh, you'll find my name on the front of the envelope."
9. A young boy wrote an essay which contained this statement: "Soap smells nice, but it tastes awful. It tastes worst of all if you get it in your eyes."

DRILL 109

Directions: Answer aloud the following questions.

1. What should you do when you are thirsty?
2. Why do we have furnaces in our homes?
3. Why do you carry an umbrella when it rains?
4. Why do we have newspapers?
5. Why do we have automobiles?
6. Why do we have policemen?
7. Why do we have telephones?
8. Why are windows made of glass?
9. Why do we use pot holders?
10. Why do we have refrigerators?
11. Why do we sleep?
12. Why do we use tire chains when driving in snow?
13. Why does property in town cost more than property in the country?
14. Why does the state require a person to get a temporary license before learning to drive a car?
15. What should you do if you find a stamped and addressed envelope on the sidewalk?
16. Why does the state require doctors to be licensed?

DRILL 110

Directions: Encircle the correct word.

1. Which can you hear?
    chair   radio   rug

2. Which can you smell?
    fork   perfume   door

3. Which belongs in a kitchen?
    sink   car   office

4. Which is used for writing?
    stove   closet   pencil

5. Which is used on a bed?
    dog   sheet   telephone

6. Which is part of a suit?
    screws   pants   coal

7. Which is part of a train?
    engine   corn   boat

8. Which can be used for transportation?
    coal   bicycle   bed

9. Which is part of a shoe?
    oats   sole   china

10. Which can be used for hose?
    blanket   nylon   cream

11. Which is part of an airplane?
    bus   wing   car

12. Which is green?
    air   grass   wood

© *Mary Coates Longerich 1955, 1958*

DRILL 111

Directions: Tell how these pairs are alike.

1. pen — pencil
2. airplane — bird
3. grass — flowers
4. coffee — milk
5. nickle — dime
6. car — bicycle
7. rain — snow
8. flashlight — lamp
9. sun — moon
10. newspaper — magazine

DRILL 112

Directions: Tell in what way these things are alike:

1. Gold and silver.
2. Iron and steel.
3. Airplane and boat.
4. Orange and lemon.
5. Lake and stream.
6. Nickel and dime.
7. Duck and goose.
8. Truck and motorcycle.
9. Horse and cow.
10. Magazine and newspaper.
11. Silk and nylon.
12. Meat and potatoes.
13. Corn and peas.
14. Watch and clock.
15. Man and boy.

DRILL 113

Directions (to be read to the patient by the aphasia therapist): I shall read one short phrase. Then I shall read the first word of another phrase, and you give me the final word of that incomplete phrase. For example, I shall say *fish—swim; birds* _____. Then you reply, *fly*.

1. knife — fork; sugar _____.   (cream)
2. liver — meat; beans _____.   (vegetables)
3. bee — bug; robin _____.   (bird)
4. grandfather — grandson; grandmother _____.   (granddaughter)
5. glove — hand; hat _____.   (head)
6. birds — sing; dogs _____.   (bark)
7. coffee — drink; cigar _____.   (smoke)
8. car — gasoline; refrigerator _____.   (electricity, gas)
9. wind — blows; moon _____.   (shines)
10. corn — grain; orange _____.   (fruit)
11. salmon — fish; canary _____.   (bird)
12. dinner — eat; newspaper _____.   (read)
13. husband — wife; man _____.   (woman)
14. horses — neigh; ducks _____.   (quack)
15. red — color; Ford _____.   (car)
16. day — night; morning _____.   (evening)
17. Sunday — day; January _____.   (month)
18. hear — ears; see _____.   (eyes)
19. arm — hand; leg _____.   (foot)
20. soldier — Army; sailor _____.   (Navy)

DRILL 114

Directions: Supply the correct word in the following sentences.

1. Steak is to eat as iced tea is to _____.
2. Waves are to the Navy as Wacs are to the _____.
3. TV is to livingroom as refrigerator is to _____.
4. Steel is to heavy as cotton is to _____.
5. The rug is to floor as pictures are to _____.
6. Sugar is to sweet as lemons are to _____.
7. The box is to wood as bottle is to _____.
8. Toe is to foot as finger is to _____.
9. Arm is to elbow as leg is to _____.
10. Apples are to fruit as corn is to _____.
11. Ruby is to red as coal is to _____.
12. New York is to U.S. as London is to _____.
13. North is to south as east is to _____.
14. Hot is to cold as winter is to _____.
15. Fork is to knife as cup is to _____.
16. Three sides are to triangle as four sides are to _____.
17. Boy is to girl as male is to _____.
18. Smooth is to rough as soft is to _____.
19. Mayor is to city as governor is to _____.
20. Client is to lawyer as patient is to _____.
21. Tailor is to clothes as baker is to _____.
22. Day is to week as month is to _____.
23. Hen is to rooster as woman is to _____.
24. Up is to down as beginning is to _____.
25. Sleep is to bed as sit is to _____.

DRILL 115

Directions: Read the first two words on each line and observe the relationship which exists between each word group. Encircle the word in the parentheses which is related in a similar way to the third word.

1. Bull — dog; Persian (goat, cat, breed)
2. Winter — November; summer (lakes, flowers, August)
3. Jane — Bob; woman (lady, doctor, man)
4. Feathers — bird; fur (robin, cat, chicken)
5. Hour — day; month (summer, seconds, year)
6. Cup — coffee; bottle (milk, lable, cap)
7. Red — stop; green (leaves, go, grass)
8. Mend — shirt; darn (socks, holes, rip)
9. Write — letter; read (story, book, aloud)
10. Market — groceries; department store (building, clothing, salesclerk)
11. Arm — finger; leg (food, toe, ankle)
12. Hungry — eat; thirsty (water, milk, drink)
13. Pencil — write; needle (thread, sharp, sew)
14. Navy — sailor; Army (march, soldier, guns)
15. Sheep — wool; fox (fur, sly, animal)
16. Fruit — apple; vegetable (green, healthy, carrot)
17. Boy — man; girl (pretty, adult, woman)
18. Good — better; bad (worse, poor, good)
19. Composer — music; painter (paint, brush, picture)
20. Cook — food; iron (hot, clothes, smooth)

DRILL 116

Directions: In the space in front of the name of each coin indicate the number of such coins you will need to answer the questions.

1. What 2 coins add up to a dollar?

    _____ Halves

    _____ Quarters

    _____ Dimes

    _____ Nickels

    _____ Pennies

2. What 2 coins add up to 15 cents?

    _____ Halves

    _____ Quarters

    _____ Dimes

    _____ Nickels

    _____ Pennies

3. What 3 coins add up to 75 cents?

    _____ Halves

    _____ Quarters

    _____ Dimes

    _____ Nickels

    _____ Pennies

4. What 3 coins add up to 16 cents?

    _____ Halves

    _____ Quarters

    _____ Dimes

    _____ Nickels

    _____ Pennies

5. What 2 coins add up to 75 cents?

    _____ Halves

    _____ Quarters

    _____ Dimes

    _____ Nickels

    _____ Pennies

6. What 3 coins add up to 25 cents?

    _____ Halves

    _____ Quarters

    _____ Dimes

    _____ Nickels

    _____ Pennies

(*continued on following page*)

DRILL 116 (cont.)

7. What 4 coins add up to 50 cents?

   _____ Halves

   _____ Quarters

   _____ Dimes

   _____ Nickels

   _____ Pennies

8. What 3 coins add up to 65 cents?

   _____ Halves

   _____ Quarters

   _____ Dimes

   _____ Nickels

   _____ Pennies

9. What 4 coins add up to 30 cents?

   _____ Halves

   _____ Quarters

   _____ Dimes

   _____ Nickels

   _____ Pennies

10. What 3 coins add up to 55 cents?

    _____ Halves

    _____ Quarters

    _____ Dimes

    _____ Nickels

    _____ Pennies

11. What 5 coins add up to 82 cents?

    _____ Halves

    _____ Quarters

    _____ Dimes

    _____ Nickels

    _____ Pennies

12. What 5 coins add up to 51 cents?

    _____ Halves

    _____ Quarters

    _____ Dimes

    _____ Nickels

    _____ Pennies

© Mary Coates Longerich 1955, 1958

DRILL 117

Directions: Read the numbers. Study the sequence; then write the numbers that should come next in the spaces.

1.	5	6	7	8	9	_____	_____
2.	5	10	15	20	25	_____	_____
3.	11	10	9	8	7	_____	_____
4.	15	18	21	24	27	_____	_____
5.	80	70	60	50	40	_____	_____
6.	4	8	12	16	20	_____	_____
7.	12	14	16	18	20	_____	_____
8.	9	18	27	36	45	_____	_____
9.	21	18	15	12	9	_____	_____
10.	1	3	5	7	9	_____	_____
11.	2	4	8	16	32	64	_____	_____
12.	1	2	4	7	11	16	_____	_____
13.	45	44	42	39	35	30	_____	_____
14.	4	6	10	12	16	18	_____	_____
15.	10	5	15	10	20	15	_____	_____

DRILL 118

Directions: Make a cross with your pen or pencil in this space _____ and encircle the longer of these two words: *house, home.* If a cow is smaller than a rat, make a cross here _____ , but if it is not, proceed with the next question and tell what is the largest state in the United States _____ . If Alaska is a part of the United States, draw a line through your last answer; but if it is not, answer this question: How many legs does a cow have? _____ . Give a wrong answer to this next question. How many feet does a person have? _____ . Look at these next two words: *up, down*; if $3 \times 7 = 21$, write the shorter word here _____ . If October comes after September make a cross here _____ , but if it does not, make a dash here _____ . Answer this question: Do horses have horns? _____ . Write nothing after this question: $9 \times 10 =$ _____ . Then, if dogs can sneeze, write a number between 3 and 5 _____ . Now write your first name _____ .

DRILL 119

Directions: Draw a circle with your pencil in this space _____. If diamonds are less plentiful than sea shells, put a cross here _____. If automobiles are made of cotton, write the word *cotton* here _____. If they are not, leave this space blank _____. If December comes after November, write the date of New Year's Day here _____. If you think that a pond is a piece of land, draw a circle here _____; but if it is not, leave this space blank _____. If 6 × 8 = 46, write the shortest of the two words *come* and *go* in this space _____; if 6 × 8 does not equal 46, then put a cross here _____. If a mouse is bigger than a cat, draw a circle in this space _____. If mules have tails, put a dash here _____; if they do not, solve this problem 8 × 10 = _____. After you have answered these questions, write the date here _____. If it is now June, write your last name here _____.

DRILL 120

Directions: Put a check in the blank which correctly completes the sentence.

1. The Fourth of July is a holiday in _____ Mexico, _____ Africa, _____ United States.

2. The Rocky Mountains are in _____ Maine, _____ Florida, _____ Colorado.

3. The sun rises in the _____ east, _____ west, _____ south.

4. The Mississippi River flows into the _____ Atlantic Ocean, _____ Pacific Ocean, _____ Gulf of Mexico.

5. Woodrow Wilson was a former _____ Governor of Iowa, _____ President of the United States, _____ Marine.

6. A canary is a _____ cat, _____ rat, _____ bird.

7. Tom Sawyer is the name of a _____ man, _____ book, _____ monument.

8. Louisiana is next to _____ Mexico, _____ New York, _____ Mississippi.

9. Thanksgiving is in _____ October, _____ February, _____ November.

10. Maltese is a type of _____ bird, _____ cat, _____ dog.

11. Sacramento is the capital of _____ Florida, _____ California, _____ Arizona.

12. The largest state in the Union is _____ California, _____ New York, _____ Texas.

13. Hawaii belongs to _____ United States, _____ England, _____ Japan.

(continued on following page)

© Mary Coates Longerich 1955, 1958

DRILL 120 (cont.)

14. William Shakespeare was a _____ composer, _____ artist, _____ writer.

15. Mardi Gras is a festival held in _____ New York, _____ New Orleans, _____ Kansas City.

DRILL 121

Directions (to be read to the patient by the aphasia therapist): Check the phrase which will complete each of the following sentences.

1. The National Anthem is
    a. The Star Spangled Banner
    b. Yankee Doodle
    c. God Bless America

2. The Pilgrims landed at
    a. Pearl Harbor
    b. Plymouth Rock
    c. San Francisco

3. The Lone Star State is
    a. Florida
    b. Texas
    c. California

4. Thomas Edison invented the
    a. Electric light
    b. Radio
    c. Television

5. Pennsylvania was named for
    a. The Pennsylvania Railroad
    b. William Penn
    c. A fountain pen

6. George Washington was known as
    a. The Father of His Country
    b. Old Ironsides
    c. F.D.R.

7. Alexander Graham Bell invented
    a. The lightning rod
    b. The telephone
    c. The steam engine

8. The Wright Brothers invented
    a. The airplane
    b. The telegraph
    c. The cotton gin

9. The largest city west of the Mississippi River is
    a. Denver, Colorado
    b. Salt Lake City, Utah
    c. Los Angeles, California

10. The Gettysburg Address was delivered by
    a. Abraham Lincoln
    b. Herbert Hoover
    c. Dwight D. Eisenhower

11. Mexico borders on
    a. Florida
    b. Texas
    c. Louisiana

12. The Fourth of July is a holiday in
    a. Mexico
    b. England
    c. The United States

© Mary Coates Longerich 1955, 1958

DRILL 122

Directions: Read the following words and tell if they are things you can do or things you can smell. Place each word in the appropriate part of the box.

roses	sing	drink	swim
walk	ride	go	vinegar
perfume	skunk	onions	laugh
run	eat	dance	ammonia
	smile	cologne	

DO	SMELL

DRILL 123

Directions: Read the following words. Then place each of them in the appropriate column.

yesterday	quickly	here	extremely
very	now	soon	noontime
quite	late	Tuesday	outdoors
today	outside	inside	below
up	there	rather	occasionally

HOW	WHEN	WHERE